PRAISE FOR PUNISH THE MACHINE!

Thank goodness we are leaving the age of information and entering the age of Intelligence in health care. To be able to really deliver value in our effort to transform health care requires us to look at new and innovative ways to manage data and turn it into insights at the very point of care. One of the huge challenges in health care informatics has been the ability to deal with the sheer variety and volume of disparate health care data and the increasing need to derive clarity and value. Punish the Machine! The Promise of Artificial Intelligence in Health Care *is a must read for physician leaders, health executives, clinical researchers, public health officials, data scientists and software engineers seeking to understand this innovation in the information revolution in health care. It provides a very readable, detailed introduction of artificial intelligence.*

DR. PAUL GRUNDY
Global Director of Healthcare Transformation, HealthTeamWorks
Founding President, Patient Centered Primary Care Collaborative
Past Chief Medical Officer and Global Director of Healthcare
Transformation, IBM

Uli Chettipally has written a must-read book for anyone involved in health care. Artificial intelligence will be changing the way we practice medicine, and Dr. Chettipally is a leader in helping clinicians effortlessly obtain cutting edge clinical research guidelines to improve patient care. Read this book and learn from one of the best.

KAREN MURRELL, MD, MBA
Chair, Emergency Medicine, The Permanente Medical Group

There is no question that health care is transforming to individual accountability where personalized and preventative medicine will take a much larger role. Individuals will learn to rely less on a broken health care delivery model which relies on health plans with conflicting incentives. This book showcases the importance of data, information and knowledge in the process of transitioning to a model requiring enhanced self-accountability. Artificial intelligence is one of the nine steps to financial recovery listed at Health-Wealth.com, and is a no-brainer when it comes to the future of health care.

DR. JOSH LUKE
Futurist
Hospital CEO
Two-time Amazon #1 Best Selling Author
Faculty, University of Southern California

Uli Chettipally's new book, Punish the Machine!, *covers so much more than just artificial intelligence and machine learning. It is a primer on what is wrong with American medicine and a guide to how to fix it. Artfully written, with compelling examples, this is a must-read for anyone interested in where health care has been and where it is going in the future.*

PATRICIA SALBER, MD, MBA
CEO, Founder, and Editor-in-Chief, The Doctor Weighs In

Dr. Chettipally has written an insightful overview of the power artificial intelligence can bring to medical practice. He offers clear examples of what is possible for the patient, the doctor and businesses, as well as providing insights into the challenges of implementation. Ultimately, as our nation moves from fee-for-service to pay-for-value and implements technology including video, voice recognition and wearable devices, AI will be as valuable and prevalent in the future as the stethoscope was in the past.

DR. ROBERT PEARL
Bestselling Author of *Mistreated: Why We Think We're Getting Good Health Care and Why We're Usually Wrong*
Health Care Contributor, Forbes
Past Executive Director and CEO, The Permanente Medical Group

PUNISH
THE
MACHINE!

Uli K. Chettipally, MD, MPH

PUNISH THE **MACHINE!**

The Promise of Artificial Intelligence in Health Care

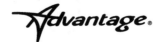

Published by Advantage, Charleston, South Carolina.
Member of Advantage Media Group.

ADVANTAGE is a registered trademark, and the Advantage colophon is a trademark of Advantage Media Group, Inc.

Printed in the United States of America.

10 9 8 7 6 5 4 3 2 1

ISBN: 978-1-59932-944-4
LCCN: 2018967226

Cover design by Mary Hamilton.
Interior design by Carly Blake.

This publication is designed to provide accurate and authoritative information in regard to the subject matter covered. It is sold with the understanding that the publisher is not engaged in rendering legal, accounting, or other professional services. If legal advice or other expert assistance is required, the services of a competent professional person should be sought.

Advantage Media Group is proud to be a part of the Tree Neutral® program. Tree Neutral offsets the number of trees consumed in the production and printing of this book by taking proactive steps such as planting trees in direct proportion to the number of trees used to print books. To learn more about Tree Neutral, please visit **www.treeneutral.com**.

Advantage Media Group is a publisher of business, self-improvement, and professional development books and online learning. We help entrepreneurs, business leaders, and professionals share their Stories, Passion, and Knowledge to help others Learn & Grow. Do you have a manuscript or book idea that you would like us to consider for publishing? Please visit **advantagefamily.com** or call **1.866.775.1696**.

To Siri, Vamsi, and Kiran and their healthy future.

To Swathi—without your encouragement,
this work would not have been possible.

TABLE OF CONTENTS

FOREWORD

Mary Shelley's book, *Frankenstein; or, The Modern Prometheus* was published over two hundred years ago in 1818.

Now, once again, we are grappling with the impact of an endless stream of technologies that are changing how we live, work and play. One is data and artificial intelligence (AI)—the theory and development of computer systems able to perform tasks that normally require human intelligence, such as visual perception, speech recognition, decision-making, and translation between languages.

All industries, including health care, are fighting to win the fourth industrial revolution. It is an economic engine driven by the confluence of man, machines, and materials that are changing the future of work, society, and how we should control the intended and unintended consequences of science and technology on people. We now live in a world of collective cyber intelligence that has brought us robots, chat bots, and driverless cars.

In this book, Dr. Chettipally, an accomplished clinician, researcher, teacher, and leader in the use of artificial intelligence in medicine, sets out to make this transformation clear to the average patient. He explains the technology and the potential intended and unintended consequences that should make us take pause.

Much like our inability to predict the impact of the iPhone when it was released on June 29th, 2007, no one will be able to predict the full impact of artificial intelligence. However, artificial intelligence has become "like the new electricity" and is being used in virtually every industry to drive growth, and hopefully, scale the potential of humans, not replace them.

Punish the Machine: The Promise of Artificial Intelligence in Health Care is a useful guide to helping you and your children understand what's going on during your next doctor visit or hospitalization and how AI is helping with how health care professionals and administrators are using it to take care of you cut through the hype. Be sure to read this book before your next medical appointment.

ARLEN MEYERS, MD, MBA

President and CEO, Society of Physician Entrepreneurs
Director, Biomedical Entrepreneurship Program, University of Colorado
Denver Business School

PREFACE

Writing about artificial intelligence is a daunting task. The subject is deep and the field is growing at a fast pace. The use cases for this technology are rapidly proliferating. What one has written today can become obsolete very quickly. The amount of innovation and brain power that is being put into play is tremendous. Some of the best minds are engaged in solving the toughest problems our society is facing today.

It is important for me to say what this book is and is not about.

This book is not a technical or engineering book about artificial intelligence. It is not a text book for learners of data science nor the craft of machine learning. It is not a research compendium nor a review of the studies that are out there.

This book is written for a broad audience in the health care and technology fields about the potential of this technology in health care. It is meant to inspire the leaders in these fields to explore possibilities. It is written to cast a vision for the future, where this technology could solve the toughest problems we are facing in health care. This book is written to stimulate thinking in people's minds of the possibility of a bright and healthy future for humankind.

CHAPTER 1

The Promise of Technology

In the classic Western *The Magnificent Seven*, a small village of peace-loving and naïve people hires a crew of seven gunfighters to protect them from the marauding bandits who have been terrorizing them. Now, I haven't seen this movie in probably forty years, but one scene still sticks with me. In it, one of the gunfighters, played by Charles Bronson, is training one of the villagers to shoot a rifle. He keeps trying, but the villager just doesn't get it. At one point, Bronson's character loses his patience, takes the gun away from the villager, and says, "I'll tell you what: don't shoot the gun. Take the gun like this, and you use it like a club. All right?" He holds the gun by the barrel and demonstrates hitting someone over the head with the butt of the gun.

This is a simple moment of comedy in a classic film, but it stuck with me, and I think it illustrates something important. A gun is a sophisticated weapon, but because of hurdles against using it properly and to fullest effect, the villager is encouraged to use it as a crude instrument. I think this reflects something that often happens with new technologies: because they are unfamiliar, we use them for much simpler tasks than what they are designed for and so fail to use them to their full potential.

This is exactly the case with information technology (IT) in health care today. While IT can be very sophisticated technology that could be used to great effect in clinical settings, we are only using it as a very blunt instrument, and it is not delivering the results we want.

With this book I hope to push us in the direction of using IT and artificial intelligence (AI) in the right way—the way it's supposed to be used to produce the most impact.

Wasted Technology

Health care, of course, is a hot topic, mainly because it is rife with problems, particularly in the United States, which spends nearly 20 percent of GDP on it.[1] Health care suffers from consistently climbing costs, which will continue to climb even though the quality we get in return is very poor. In other words, the 20 percent of GDP we are spending on health care is being spent very poorly. In addition, physicians themselves face very high levels of burnout. Furthermore, based on both statistical evidence and my own anecdotal experience,[2] I can affirm that 50 percent of what physicians do in a typical US clinical

---

1   "National Health Expenditure Projections 2017–2026," Centers for Medicare and Medicaid Services, https://www.cms.gov/Research-Statistics-Data-and-Systems/Statistics-Trends-and-Reports/NationalHealthExpendData/Downloads/ForecastSummary.pdf.

2   Elizabeth A. McGlynn et al., "The Quality of Health Care Delivered to Adults in the United States," *New England Journal of Medicine* 348, no. 26 (June 26, 2003): 2635–2645, https://doi.org/10.1056/NEJMsa022615.

practice is unnecessary, ineffective, or dangerous. In what follows, I intend to show the connection among these three seemingly disparate issues: high spending on health care, physician burnout, and the delivery of low-quality patient care.

Let me begin with the obvious: we are dealing with a massive amount of waste. One of the problems that cause waste is that physicians are not given the right tools. The technological tools that they do have, such as the electronic health record (EHR), are being used as very blunt instruments. While EHRs could be used in connection with AI to improve quality, lower costs, unburden physicians, and guide clinical decision making, they are instead used for three simple, crude reasons, none of which has to do with improving quality, and which mostly concern mitigating risk.

REIMBURSEMENT

First, the EHR, basically, is a billing tool. Doctors must document everything they do in the EHR so they will be able to bill for the service. The documentation allows them to list all the procedures they performed and what needs to be paid for. If physicians don't document fully, they risk not getting paid.

Let's say you went to the doctor with a sprained ankle. She might document the fact that you're alert and oriented, check your heart rate, monitor your breathing, and record several other things that are not directly related to your sprained ankle. The more boxes she can check off, the more procedures she will have reimbursed. She may have to document a certain number of factors in order to be reimbursed for taking an x-ray, so since she will get reimbursed for the x-ray, too, she will be sure to document all of those things. Whether the x-ray is actually needed in a particular case is a secondary issue.

That may sound sinister, but it is actually just the behavior that is incentivized in the current business model of fee for service health care. This helps the doctor, of course, but it does almost nothing for the patient in terms of clinical care, improved health, or positive outcomes.

LEGAL PROTECTION

Second, the EHR can be used as a legal document. Let's say there is a bad outcome, and the patient or family of the patient sues the doctor or the hospital. Then the EHR becomes a legal document intended to protect the doctor. Obviously, the lawyer is going to ask, "So what did you do for this patient?" Usually, this happens a few years after the doctor has seen the patient, and the doctor may not even remember the interaction. For that reason, doctors document as much as they possibly can on each visit in order to reduce the risk down the road of running into a legal problem and needing to account for details.

In other words, the documentation in the EHR becomes a valuable mechanism of defense in the case of bad outcomes that lead to malpractice suits; the providers—either the physicians or the hospitals—can use the medical records to defend themselves: "These are the things that we did; this is all compliant with the standard of care. Therefore, the bad outcome is not our fault." Of course, on the other side, the plaintiffs and their lawyers also have access to the record in case they need to point out where the defendant is mistaken and further care should have been provided.

Let's go back to your sprained ankle. Say the doctor took an x-ray but missed a very small fracture on the x-ray, so you sue her. The EHR will allow the doctor to report that she did her due diligence, checking on just the right factors. Perhaps there is also a record of her telling you about the risk of a small fracture, even though it is not visible on the x-ray, and advising you to follow up if the pain lasts more than a few days. Documenting that she has done her due diligence is a large part of what the doctor is doing with your EHR during your visit.

REGULATORY COMPLIANCE

Finally, there are a number of steps and actions that regulatory agencies want to make sure doctors are doing consistently: checking blood pressure and blood sugar, discussing smoking cessation with patients who smoke, and so forth. For diabetics, for instance, doctors have to make sure certain tests are done and checked off a checklist. Some of these items do reflect what needs to be done for the patient. Others have little research behind them and are therefore questionable. Still, others may have become obsolete—a fact the physician is unaware of.

All three of these EHR-related tasks—forms of risk mitigation—are important and necessary, but they are only peripherally related to the primary aim of any health care practice: the health of the patients. Many of the things doctors document, especially for legal and regulatory purposes, are not even necessary to clinical care. Even for reimbursement purposes, much of the information that payers require will not help the patient in any way. But that's what the payer wants, so the doctor does it.

Wasted Opportunity

The big thing that is missing from this picture is that EHRs are not being used to improve the quality of care that patients receive. In particular, EHRs are only used to document past and present data, not to look toward the future. The benefit of the EHR being electronic or digital is simply that it saves paper in the documentation process. The capacities of digital technology to improve care quality are not being exploited. Quite honestly, they are barely being considered.

Of course, having an electronically accessible health record has the benefit of allowing doctors to go back and look at a patient's previous encounters with the health system. Ease of accessibility also allows the EHR to provide alerts and reminders for the physician to do certain things or not do certain things. For example, the EHR can alert the physician to check certain lab tests in a patient with a given illness. Or it can alert the physician about certain drug interactions, based on what the patient is taking and what the doctor wants to prescribe. These are all good things.

However, the EHR is not being used in such a way that the doctor can ask, "Okay, for the last one hundred patients with this symptom, I did this; what have the outcomes been? How would it change the outcome if I were to do something else? Should I rely on drug A or drug B to manage this symptom? Is there something else I am missing? Is there something else I should be doing? Is the procedure that I'm doing actually benefitting the patients? How does this outcomes information I have from the previous one hundred patients change the way I treat my next patient with the same problem?" The EHR by itself is silent on all of these clinical decision-making questions. It's not just that much of the information doctors are required to enter is totally irrelevant to patient care; it's that a lot of truly relevant information is not even required to be documented and is therefore left unaddressed.

Let's return once more to your sprained ankle. Is there clinical information that needs to be collected in order to predict the likelihood of a fracture? Is there information that will help reduce the need for an x-ray to avoid unnecessary exposure to radiation? Some variables might affect the likelihood of you having a small fracture.

So the doctor could have identified that risk more accurately had she had information about those variables. Also, an analysis of her records could show that one course of treatment for certain cases of a sprained ankle would work better than another. Given these factors, she might be able to tell you whether heat or cold would be more effective for treatment. As it stands with EHRs, though, there is no way to access this information. Even if your doctor has been treating sprained ankles for years, she has no rigorous scientific basis for recommending the best course of treatment for a particular case.

Let's say a physician sees patients with arthritis on a daily basis, so that, by the end of the year, she has seen roughly five hundred patients, all with the same problem. On the one hand, we would expect the care that the most recent patient receives would be the same as the first, After all, it's the same problem. On the other hand, the doctor has built up a year's worth of experience and five hundred patients' worth of information. It should be possible for the doctor to make improvements to the care she is offering on the basis of this experience and data.

Of course, as time progresses after physicians first join a practice or start their own, clinical decision making is likely to improve. This occurs at the level of human performance improvement: the brain starts to learn, to recognize patterns, and make appropriate decisions, but the limits to this improvement are the same as the limits to any human brain. It's true that experience allows the doctor to recommend one treatment over another, but it's strange that this accumulated experience—from patient one to patient five hundred, or five thousand—doesn't necessarily change the physician's practice in any substantial way.

The fact that the care of the five-hundredth patient is likely not very different from that of the first is something we ought to question. The fact that physicians may have seen hundreds of patients in between the first and the most recent does not help them in any meaningful way. They have *no scientific way* of tracking and understanding whether what they are doing is helping, and to what extent. It might even be impossible for them to know which components of a given treatment are the ones that are having a positive effect and which others may be useless, or worse, negatively affect outcomes. Clinical practice does not allow for studying this, so there is no way to know with any certainty!

As I hinted at before, a lot of the information that could be used to predict outcomes and guide treatment is not required to be entered into the EHR, which is therefore unlikely to capture the information that would affect outcomes and treatment. Even worse, we may not yet know precisely which information is relevant for us to capture and document were we to employ the EHR as a means of predicting outcomes.

My point is this: doctors end up entering the minimum required amount of information in order to save time as much as possible. Clinically relevant information may be left out because doctors are documenting so many other things that the relevant information becomes secondary. Even if relevant information *is* entered into the EHR, doctors still don't have the tools at their disposal to *use* that information for improving patient care. As EHRs are currently used, the information just sits there, unable to answer any questions. With the right technology, though, we can go beyond the limits of a given human brain and have the equivalent of one thousand brains working on a question simultaneously. This could help lead us to better clinical decisions and, eventually, better outcomes for patients.

AI is a tool that would make it possible to answer some of these questions based solely on current EHR information, but this possibility is not being taken advantage of. Doctors could use the information in the EHR in combination with AI's ability to search, refine, and manipulate data to figure out the best ways of caring for their patients.

Using EHRs as blunt instruments diminishes the quality of care, of course, but it is also the reason so many doctors are burned out. The physician's job is to provide care and make the patient healthier. However, what physicians spend a great deal of their time and effort doing—in some cases, most of their time and effort—is recording various items for the three purposes we discussed earlier: reimbursement, regulation, and medicolegal documentation. The primary purpose of delivering care has fallen by the wayside, or at least to the fourth position on the list. Ultimately, doctors feel dissatisfied, frustrated, and overworked because all these little things add up and consume a lot of time. In place of focusing on helping patients, physicians are focused primarily on entering data into the EHR. For every hour physicians provide direct clinical face time to patients, nearly two additional hours are spent on EHR and desk work during the clinic day. Physicians spend another one to two hours of personal time each night doing additional computer and other clerical work.[3] Data entry minimizes the role of the physician to documentation at the expense of the roles of teaching and healing.

Over time, the amount of information physicians have to include to satisfy all of these requirements keeps growing and increasing their burden, so they are spending more and more time interacting with EHRs and less and less time interacting with patients. We should not be surprised that surveys of burned-out doctors show EHRs as the number-one reason for burnout. Instead of being seen as a useful tool, the records currently are felt to be a burden. Insofar as EHRs are not tied to quality patient outcomes, their primary purpose is not

---

3   C. Sinsky et al., "Allocation of Physician Time in Ambulatory Practice: A Time and Motion Study in 4 Specialties," *Annals of Internal Medicine* 165, no. 11 (December 6, 2016): 753–760, https://doi.org/10.7326/M16-0961.

being met. This frustrates doctors and makes them dissatisfied with their work.[4] The job that was supposed to center on caring for people becomes a very mundane and mechanical process for the purpose of satisfying non-clinical goals. A lot of the time, this critical work of determining what's going on with a patient is work that goes home with the physician. As you can imagine, a chronic overload of work leads to missing out on social and family life and affects a doctor's emotional and mental health. We see more and more mental health issues in doctors, including higher rates of substance abuse and suicide compared to the rest of the population.[5]

It should be no surprise that from the patient side, the number one patient complaint about primary care is that the doctor doesn't spend enough time, let alone enough quality time, with them. The doctor is too busy entering data into EHRs. Sometimes, again, this is to the detriment of the actual care being delivered because the doctor doesn't have enough time *while in the patient's presence* to figure out what's actually going on with that particular patient.

On top of this, there are problems with the EHRs themselves: these systems have often been designed using technology that is thirty or more years old. Beyond being outdated, they are often poorly designed because EHR companies are not accountable to the end users, the doctors. Their relationship is mediated by third party buyers who do not actually use the system and make decisions based soley on other considerations. Even government incentives, although given to health care entities to help them financially, do not help with the

---

4   Tait D. Shanafelt et al., "Relationship between Clerical Burden and Characteristics of the Electronic Environment with Physician Burnout and Professional Satisfaction," Mayo Clinic Proceedings 91, no. 7 (July 2016): 836–848, https://doi. org/10.1016/j.mayocp.2016.05.007.

5   Omotola O. T'Sarumi et al., "Physician Suicide: A Silent Epidemic," Poster Proceedings no. 227, American Psychiatric Association, Annual Meeting, May 5–9, 2018, New York City.

design and usability of EHRs. For these reasons, EHRs continue to be mere repositories of information; they are not yet smart technologies. Currently, they are being used for documenting care processes for the purposes of reimbursement, reduction of medicolegal risk, and regulation fulfillment.

Yet the data within them could answer questions if we were able to put questions to them. The potential of AI for clinical applications is the main focus of this book, and in later chapters I'll discuss various applications, both actual and speculative. With sophisticated AI, the electronic system that is collecting the data should be able to identify which data are relevant and need to be collected and should be able to help the physician come up with treatment or management solutions that actually help patients. For now, the EHR acts as a dump for data and gives nothing back of much clinical use.

AI Impact

Over the past two decades, the technology at the heart of AI and machine learning has progressed rapidly, and these developments have great potential for applications that would be transformative for health care. Many experts in the field are already promoting some of these applications, but their focus tends to be limited to the administrative side of things. The 2017 Accenture list of the top ten AI applications in health care, for example, includes far more administrative tasks than practices that might apply to direct clinical care and practice.[6]

---

6   Matt Collier, Richard Fu, and Lucy Yin, "Artificial Intelligence: Health Care's New Nervous System," Accenture, 2017, https://www.accenture.com/t20171215T032059Z__w__/us-en/_acnmedia/PDF-49/Accenture-Health-Artificial-Intelligence.pdf#zoom=50.

The clinical setting, however, is where AI can have the most disruptive impact in terms of both health outcomes and lowered costs. AI can not only make predictions but also provide guidance in prevention, diagnosis, treatment, and other functions of clinical decision making. In the clinical setting, AI is potentially paradigm changing. More than 95 percent of physicians already gather data on their patients via EHRs, which means there is a treasure trove of data out there waiting to be explored and exploited.

The availability of this data, *together with AI technology*, can lead to an explosion in the kind of medical knowledge that doctors draw on in clinical decision making. In the past, medical knowledge has been achieved by what we all recognize as the traditional scientific method: a research question is formulated, a hypothesis is developed, and data is gathered from a sample study population and compared to controls in order to confirm or refute the hypothesis. In the health care sphere, this data gathering step occurs by means of clinical trials, which are, by necessity, limited to small portions of the population in very restricted conditions.

I'll discuss this at greater length later but let me put the idea in your head now that AI allows us to reverse the order of this process. In cases where the EHR is well utilized for record keeping, we have already gathered data from a sizable portion of the population. So, we can begin by presenting our questions to this already existing data set. The data manipulation and pattern recognition capabilities of AI can then be employed to generate and confirm answers to real life questions and with real-time application for current patients.

AI's big advantage over the limitations of clinical trials is that its data set can be drawn from the records of many thousands, potentially millions, of people, as opposed to a clinical trial that has to operate with a much smaller and less random population. Because clinical trials narrow their focus to a small subset of variables in a fixed period of time, they end up taking a snapshot of one moment out of the life of each subject, including only those characteristics researchers identify as potentially relevant. AI, on the other hand, can accommodate a much bigger and richer picture of a patient's entire life, taking into account any and all data points that have ever been gathered on that subject, including where patients live, what they eat, their socioeconomic status, their preferred mode of transportation, and so on. Health care professionals widely recognize that all of these things, including behavioral and social determinants of health, comprise risk factors, but this recognition is not reflected in the structure of clinical trials and, many times, it's also not reflected in their specific content. AI allows us to determine the weight of these various risk factors and use that knowledge to mitigate risks in the cases of specific patients. In combination with EHR data, AI can directly inform the actual practice of medicine at the clinical level, making use of the data that is constantly being collected to improve patient outcomes, and it can help drastically reduce health care costs. AI methodologies have the advantage of studying patients in the real-world setting rather than in a more sterile, academic clinical trial setting.[7]

The rest of this book is devoted to showing the promise of the application of AI in various clinical settings. From the broadest point of view, AI can lead to improvements in care, improved health, economic benefits, and a more effective health care system. More specifically, the application of AI in the clinical setting has potential benefits for three primary stakeholders.

---

7   Alvin Rajkomar et al., "Scalable and accurate deep learning with electronic health records," npj Digital Medicine 1, no. 18 (May 2018): https://doi.org/10.1038/s41746-018-0029-1.

PATIENTS

For patients, it's simple: better health outcomes will result from getting treatments that work. Getting the right treatment right away has a few advantages. First, patients are likely to get better faster, since they will not have to go through the trial and error process. Second, adverse reactions to treatment will decrease because appropriate treatments are identified before treatment begins. Also, the number of treatment failures will decrease. Because patients *won't* be getting treatments that *won't* work, the cost of care will be lower. So, the part of the bill that patients must foot, out of pocket or indirectly through their employers or the government, will be lower as well. For patients subscribing to high-deductible health plans, this change would be significant, given that out-of-pocket expenditures keep rising at a much faster rate than individual incomes and faster than the economy as a whole.[8]

DOCTORS

AI is not a threat to doctors. Rather, it will help them by lightening their cognitive burdens and their workloads. They will be better equipped to act on accurate risk calculations, instead of having to perform the calculations themselves. Since humans are not as accurate in making these estimations as machines are, doctors can feel relief that the care they're providing is less risky and more likely immediately beneficial to the patient. They will be able to devote their time to doing things that drive value for their patients and give meaning to their practice. Knowing that whatever they are doing is benefiting their patients will decrease the frustration and burnout that is so prevalent among them now. They will be working smart, not hard.

---

8   Les Masterson, "Out-of-Pocket Health Care Costs up 11% in 2017," Healthcare Dive brief, March 7, 2018, https://www.healthcaredive.com/news/out-of-pocket-health care-costs-up-11-in-2017/518537.

One quick example: new AI tools are coming on the market that will help physicians spend less time doing documentation and entering data manually and more time talking with the patient, interacting with the patient, understanding the patient's situation, and developing empathy for the patient's circumstances. To the extent that these new tools will also help mitigate and decrease the potential for bad outcomes, the guiding worry about malpractice should decrease as well.

COMPANIES AND ORGANIZATIONS

Finally, cost savings benefiting the bottom line are a key factor that should appeal to business leaders and employers. For providers, AI offers an accurate risk assessment and cost-benefit analysis tool for treatment options. If companies are able to decrease costs and provide care more efficiently, they will be financially rewarded. Their customer service would also improve insofar as patients would feel heard and find interacting with the system pleasurable rather than painful. Creating greater "stickiness" between patients and providers would benefit both. One note of caution, though: AI works best in a value-based care system rather than a volume-based care system.

In the following chapters, I discuss potential applications of AI to the clinical setting under the headings of prevention, diagnosis, and treatment. I'll provide case studies as well as my own speculations regarding each of these three main categories.

CHAPTER 2

Prevention: The Theory

There is an old story about a group of villagers gathered by the river on a pleasant afternoon. One of the villagers sees a child in the water, struggling against the current to keep from drowning. The water is flowing very fast. If the villagers don't intervene, the child is going to die.

Quickly, the villagers gather some ropes and successfully save the child from the current. Then someone sees another child, and another, and another, all of them coming down the river struggling not to drown. Two of the villagers run to get their boat to help with the rescue mission. Working with the boat and the ropes, the villagers continue to save the children. But the more children they rescue, the more children they notice coming down the river, all in mortal danger. While some villagers continue to work on getting the children out of the river, others set up a station to provide blankets and dry clothes for the rescued youth. Some work on taking care of wounds, others begin preparing hot soup for nourishment, and others set up fires for warmth and tents for shelter.

Eventually their efforts grow more advanced. Some of the villagers set up a wide net, so they can catch multiple children at once. Others work on gathering and preparing different foods for the children. Still others set up cots so that the children can rest more comfortably.

For days and months, the villagers put all their effort into successfully rescuing children from the dangerous current.

Then a wise old man from a neighboring village approaches. "Has anyone gone upstream to see what's happening there?" he asks.

The villagers were stunned. They had never considered *why* the children might be falling into the river in the first place.

One of the villagers runs upriver to investigate. What he finds is a bridge that the children must cross to fulfill their daily tasks. The bridge is dilapidated and looks to be missing some planks. The villager tells the children to stop using the bridge.

And just like that, the children stop coming down the river to the rescue stations that the villagers had set up below.

In this story, the villagers do a fine job of coordinating their efforts to save the young children who are threatened with drowning. But they do not consider the possibility of stopping the children from falling into the river in the first place.

That possibility is called prevention. Promoting prevention is a physician's duty, venerated as part of the Hippocratic Oath.

If we can figure out why patients are getting sick with a specific problem or specific diagnosis, we can go upstream and try to prevent that problem from happening. The data we collect, combined with the use of AI tools can help us figure out why specific problems and diagnoses arose in the first place so that we can try to stop them from happening at all or, at a minimum, decrease the likelihood of them happening.

There is a big difference between prevention and our current practices in clinical care. For one thing, if you take care of patients downstream, as we do now, there is no reduction in the actual number of people suffering from preventable illnesses. Certainly, the sooner a cancerous tumor is detected, the better the possibility of healing and extending a life. But it would be even better to detect the cancer *before it develops*. If you can identify and treat the risk factors, you can decrease the actual number of incidents of cancer. Additionally, the costs to organizations and patients go up exponentially when downstream treatment is the norm. Prevention has been shown to be much cheaper than treatment and cure. It's cheaper to prevent a cancerous tumor from developing than to operate on an already growing tumor, or using chemotherapy and radiation therapies in the later stages.

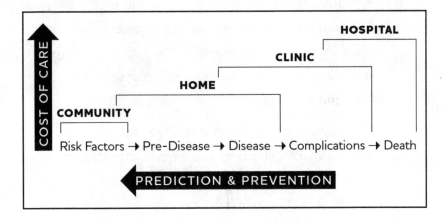

Kaiser Permanente is a good model of how focusing on prevention can help reduce health problems and diseases. A recent study found that between 2000 and 2015, heart disease death rates among adults aged forty-five to sixty-five fell by 48.3 percent in 3.2 million Kaiser Permanente Northern California members compared to a 23.6 percent decline nationwide. Stroke-related deaths for the same age group fell by 55.8 percent among Kaiser Permanente members, compared to a nationwide drop of 26.0 percent.[9] The company achieved these reductions by treating associated problems: diabetes, high blood pressure, high cholesterol, and smoking. By aggressively working on those four risk factors, the organization has been able to decrease downstream morbidity and mortality in its patient population.

Focusing clinical care on prevention would benefit all three of the stakeholders we're discussing in this book.

1. Doctors will be able to consider predictors of patient health rather than respond only to sickness. This would help them get hold of current health problems and prevent additional and more dangerous problems farther down the line.

2. Companies that focus on prevention will be the financial winners in the long run, spending less on expensive downstream care and improving their bottom line. Currently, companies spend a huge amount on health care. For some, it is the number-one cost.

3. Most importantly, patients would get better-quality care. One clear marker of quality care would be the elimination of unnecessary treatments, procedures, and surgeries. Another would be the ability to find the best medications more quickly. Still another would be the decrease in patients' future risks.

The greater our predictive abilities, the better the health outcomes of patients. Patients could stay healthy longer and live longer. Their disease burden could be lessened.

---

9   S. Sidney et al., "Comparative Trends in Health Disease, Stroke, and All-Cause Mortality in the United States and a Large Integrated Health Care Delivery System," *American Journal of Medicine* 131, no. 7 (July 2018): 829–836.e1, epub., April 2, 2018, doi: 10.1016/j.amjmed.2018.02.014.

Using AI as a Tool for Prevention

The best way to keep patients healthy is to gather data on outcomes from the patient population in its entirety. At least 95 percent of hospitals already have EHRs for gathering data. Even if the EHR system is not yet able to collect all the data points we need, it is a system that can easily be put to that task. Meanwhile, the current EHR system will at least help us determine and fine-tune the information we may need to collect in the future. Once we are able to determine which data are relevant to which outcomes, we will know precisely which information needs to be collected as well as which information is useless and can be dropped from the record.

As I'll point out later in this chapter, the model of health care will have to change to one that incentivizes preventive care for the sake of improving patient outcomes. Because AI is put to its most important use in health care by helping to predict and prevent illnesses, we will need to commit to a different business model to invest in the potentialities of AI. The benefits of doing so will be good for patients, physicians, and companies. First, though, let's quickly consider one example of AI's current use.

AI has already been used successfully with EHRs at New York University's Langone School of Medicine. A research team there used AI to perform multiple classification tasks on patient data taken from many different sources and collected over a long period of time. The researchers did this to see if AI could help predict a number of significant problems, including severe kidney disease.[10]

---

10 Narges Razavian, Jake Marcus and David Sontag, "Multi-task Prediction of Disease Onsets from Longitudinal Lab Tests," Cornell University Library, presented at 2016 Machine Learning and Healthcare conference (MLHC 2016), Los Angeles, CA.

Imagine the benefit of being able to predict, for example, who is likely to develop kidney disease. We could keep patients from going into kidney failure and needing dialysis. We could also prevent other risks closely associated with kidney failure—stroke, dementia, heart disease, and heart failure. At Langone, the use of AI for "deep learning" purposes helped the doctors there analyze risk factors in patients. In this instance, AI even identified relationships between kidney failure and certain health factors that doctors hadn't even considered before. The doctors at Langone are learning that using AI early on to help prevent or decrease risk factors means reaping the future benefit of less kidney failure overall. These researchers showed that AI can be a very beneficial aid when trying to figure out which patients are at risk and which interventions will help patients the most now to prevent the possibility of disease developing later on. This strategy, of course, works best when utilized in an environment where risk factors are treated aggressively.

The potential benefit to patients is enormous. But what about benefits to the health care system overall?

The Dominant Business Model

The business model of health care has traditionally been *fee for service* or *volume based*. In a fee-for-service model, health care companies, doctors, and hospitals make money when the patient is *sick*. The more tests and the more procedures, the more these groups profit. In a fee-for-service system, there is a tendency for providers to do more so that they can increase their income. As a doctor, the more days I put you in the hospital, the more money I make. The more EKGs

I do, the more money I make. The more operations I do, the more money I make.

The fee-for-service model is one of the main reasons that good patient outcomes are not a priority in our health care system. More sick people equals more "heads in beds," and sicker individuals mean a higher income per patient for doctors and hospitals. There is no system-wide incentive to keep patients healthy. There is also no incentive to avoid driving up health care costs by prescribing unnecessary medications, doing unnecessary surgeries, or keeping patients in the hospital unnecessarily.

Let's say, for example, that in order to address your chronic back pain, your doctor says that you should have back surgery. You may think, *Great! The doctor is going to fix my problem.* What you don't know is that it is very likely that surgery will not accomplish anything significant, and your pain, ultimately, will not go away. According to research, patients who had back surgery ten years previously report pain levels equal to those who did not have the surgery.[11] Back surgery may help a little in the short term or a few well selected patients, but there is little to no benefit in the longer term. Doctors keep performing back surgeries, however, because doctors and health care systems make money from them. In fact, this habit of using surgery as treatment for back pain has made back surgery the elective surgery on which people in the United States spend the most money.

This is just one example of how health care has become so expensive. Patients are usually not in a position to know which treatments and procedures will benefit them; they trust their doctors to recommend what is best. But doctors often turn a blind eye to

---

11   S. J. Atlas et al., "Long-Term Outcomes of Surgical and Nonsurgical Management of Lumbar Spinal Stenosis: 8 to 10-year results from the Maine Lumbar Spine Study," *Spine* 30, no. 8 (April 15, 2005): 936–943, https://www.ncbi.nlm.nih.gov/pubmed/15834339/.

research and other helpful information because they don't really want to know, or because the truth can harm their profit. If they were to acknowledge that back surgery doesn't really help patients, they would do fewer surgeries, which means they would make less money.

Sometimes even doctors are not in a position to tell if the treatments they offer make a difference or not. This happens when doctors don't have the data on outcomes that would enable them to see if what they're actually doing is in any way helping their patients, especially in the long term. There are a limited number of studies on back surgery, for example, and these limited studies show that back surgery is not really helping patients. If we had the ability to gather and process all the data on patient outcomes for back surgery, we could get very clear about its value, or lack thereof, for patient well-being. And I am sure the newer devices and techniques can be better evaluated.

Frankly, back surgery is not even a unique example. There are a number of procedures and treatments that are done on a regular basis that are largely useless, or that only benefit a very small portion of the cases in which they are used: tonsillectomies, adenoidectomies, hysterectomies, C-sections, joint replacements, cardiac bypass, and cardiac catheterization are just a few. These procedures make the system a lot of money, or at least they used to, but they do not really positively affect patient outcomes except in a few selected patients.

All of this is to say that the fee-for-service business model of health care is one of the biggest drivers of the growing cost of health care, and its effects are overall bad for patient outcomes. And maybe doctors, too, as they have to keep spinning their wheels to see more patients and subject them to more medical interventions as the reimbursement levels go down.

The good news is that the business model is changing, from a volume based one to a *value based* one, which rewards *outcomes*, instead of procedures, tests, and hospitalizations. In the value-based model, providers are paid fixed amounts per patient—typically on a monthly basis—for medication, hospitalization, or procedures. Whatever is left over from that fixed amount goes to the provider. Utilization of multiple services leads to loss of money, so the provider profits most when patients are healthy rather than when they are sick.

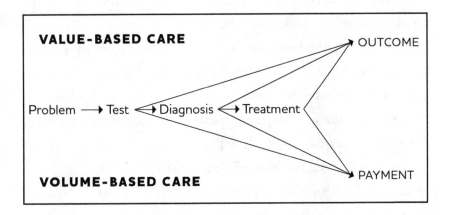

You might be surprised to learn that roughly 40 percent of organizations are working on the value-based care model.[12] The reason for the shift is that because health care costs are increasing, the payers of those costs—typically, the Centers for Medicare and Medicaid Services (CMS) and the employers who foot a big part of the insurance bill—are putting pressure on health care providers to change the model.

Even though the fee-for-service model is still dominant, value-based care is becoming more prevalent for the simple reason that the payers are increasingly unable to bear the rapidly increasing costs. Employers are switching to providers who look at outcomes,

---

12 Health Catalyst, "Hospitals Progressing Slowly toward Medicare's Goal of 50 Percent Value-Based Reimbursement by 2018," news release, May 9, 2016, https://www.healthcatalyst.com/news/hospitals-progressing-slowly-toward-medicares-goal-of-50-percent-value-based-reimbursement.

and in the new, value-based-care framework, providers *must* look at outcomes. Outcomes-based providers want to know how to keep patients healthy and eliminate waste in the form of treatment, hospitalization, medications, or devices and how to eliminate treatments and tests that are not useful for positive outcomes. In the value-based model, profit comes from positive outcomes and the elimination of wasteful procedures. In other words, focusing on prevention is one very important way to decrease the costs of care.

Until now, most health care companies haven't primarily focused on outcomes, but as the value-based system takes hold, companies are going to be increasingly forced to consider outcomes. The healthier the patient is, the *less* companies spend on treatments and therefore the more money they make. It will come to be in every company's interest to figure out the most efficient way to get the best outcomes. In this way, the provider's incentive will actually come to be more aligned with that of the patient. Patients need to be healthy; providers will focus more on making patients healthy. In the value-based system, the doctor wants patients to be healthy, the company wants patients to be healthy, and the patients want to be healthy.

The Challenges of a New Business Model

Earlier, I pointed out that reaping the benefits of AI is connected to the implementation of a value-based system of health care. Here, I want to make an even stronger point: the applications of AI that I'm advocating in this book will only work in a value-based care system, not in a fee-for-service system. This is no small matter. Let me explain.

In the case of kidney disease, we know that avoiding dialysis would save patients from illness, pain, and even debt. We also know that doing dialysis three times a week, going to the dialysis center and spending a few hours there every second or third day, is a big cost to patients and to the health care companies paying for dialysis. Why wouldn't our health care system want to avoid putting patients on dialysis?

One difficulty is that it is hard for health care organizations to see that they could profit from taking an aggressively preventive approach. Their worry is that prevention will decrease the overall size of the industry. So, there is a reluctance to adopt newer models of care, especially value-based models. This reluctance motivates political campaigning by organizations that want to keep the status quo. There is significant political opposition to the idea of value-based, preventive care because organizations believe that their piece of the pie will shrink should value-based care be fully implemented.

But as the cost of care keeps going up, a shift to value-based care is going to be inevitable. The cost of health care for American companies is already a huge burden on the economy. Those costs will also become a competitive disadvantage for American companies, as they will, eventually, lose out to competition from other countries, where health care costs are lower. The movement of health care out of the United States would be similar to the movement of jobs out of the United States. We've seen that it's cheaper to hire labor outside the United States in part because benefit packages are much smaller in other countries. Health care is the biggest benefit that US employers pay. As employers become more and more burdened with health care costs, they will have to face the issue of offering value-based care.

I mentioned earlier that organizations of varying sizes are shifting to value-based care and are coming up with programs in which patients pay a fixed monthly cost and the provider takes care of everything that happens to them. Relatively recently, the CMS launched model organizations such as the accountable care organization (ACO) and the patient-centered medical home (PCMH). These two types of organization deliver treatment in collaboration with primary care. This arrangement helps patients get the care they need in a timely fashion, in a place they're familiar with, and in a way that they can most easily understand. These models were designed to reduce costs, mainly through decreased emergency department use and decreased in-patient hospital admissions. ACOs and PCMHs make sure all the patients' needs are met and that they're watched carefully and taken care of at home without the need for hospitalizations. In these organizations, problems are tackled early on. An ACO, for example, is responsible for every aspect of care for a single patient. Reimbursements are tied to reduction in the total cost of care for all the patients served.

Another means of funding value-based care is payment bundling. In other words, all the charges surrounding a single health event aren't separated into payments to hospitals, physicians, nursing homes, testing and treatment facilities, and the like. Instead, everything is bundled into one payment based on the expected costs for a particular care event. That is yet another way of restricting how much each episode of illness will cost payers and of attempting to reduce health care costs overall. Still, another payment system that is compatible with value-based care is the pay-for-performance system, or value-based purchasing, which rewards health care providers for good patient outcomes and penalizes them for poor ones.

My overall point here is that *there are already payment models that are compatible with value-based care.* Ideally, in a mature, value-based health care system, one organization takes care of all of a given patient's needs. One organization is responsible for everything that happens to that patient and is also responsible for the entire cost of that patient's care.

Opponents of the value-based care model might argue that if a patient does not stay within a particular system for long enough, that system will lose money. This is true. The biggest challenge that health care companies face by focusing on prevention is that it is likely to take a while for them to reap profits from preventive care. This can make health care organizations reluctant to take on the proposed model; they feel they'd be doing all this extra work for no profit.

I think there is a reasonable response to these opponents. The incentive for having strong prevention and prediction programs is to have "sticky" patients, to create strong relationships and keep engaging patients on a regular basis. AI can help with this aspect of customer service by generating preventive health care plans that entice patients to stay. If the idea is to keep the patient in the system long enough for everyone—patients and companies—to reap the benefits of preventive care, then AI can be used to help retain members within the system and keep them happy. A solid EHR and a strong customer service focus might yield good practices such as sending patients regular health reminders, tracking patient health and fitness goals in real time, motivating patients daily, and tracking their overall status. Health care practitioners could contact patients to tell them, for example, that they're doing everything right, but their cholesterol is still too high, which they need to fix to decrease their risk of heart attack. Analyzing a patient's status and keeping the patient on track to becoming and staying healthy would go a long way toward keeping patients loyal to their care providers.

I would argue that it is a good thing for companies to improve patient retention by better meeting patient needs and by helping patients see the benefit of their membership in the organization. Convenience, quality, regularity and reliability of care, actual health outcomes—all these things that are part of the transition to value-based care—are things that companies should always prioritize.

The bottom line is that the more satisfied patients are, the longer they'll stay within the system. The longer they stay within the system, the more benefits the system will gain from its prevention efforts.

CHAPTER 3

Prevention: The Application

At the start of chapter 2, I mentioned the use of AI tools in clinical practice to help prevent heart disease. In this chapter, I am going to delve deeper into that example to show just how that process works. I will keep my focus in this chapter on the use of AI in *preventive* care.

Heart disease is the number-one cause of death in the United States.[13] Although we refer primarily to heart disease or cardiovascular disease, similar risk factors also affect the brain and the kidneys. Currently, some of the best-known risk factors for heart disease are older age, smoking, diabetes, high cholesterol, and high blood pressure. Others are an unhealthy diet, obesity, physical inactivity, and a family history of the disease. These core risk factors are regularly reviewed for accuracy and have been set into guidelines by the American College of

---

13   National Center for Health Statistics, *Deaths: Leading Causes for 2016*, National Vital Statistics Reports 67, no. 6 (July 26, 2018), https://www.cdc.gov/nchs/fastats/leading-causes-of-death.htm.

Cardiology (ACC) and the American Heart Association (AHA).

The primary thing that happens in a body suffering from cardiovascular disease is that the blood vessels narrow. This decreases the blood supply to vital organs. If that decrease happens suddenly, it might cause either a heart attack or a stroke. Under other circumstances, the narrowing of vessels could end up cutting off circulation to the legs, called limb ischemia, as a result of what we call peripheral vascular disease. Kidney failure can also be related to vascular disease as a risk factor.

In sum, the narrowing of the blood vessels potentially affects a lot of organs—the heart, brain, kidneys—as well as limbs. When we treat the risk factors for heart disease, all of these other diseases and health problems can also be prevented because the blood vessels are common to them all. The heart, brain, and kidney are vital organs. Without them, a person cannot live. But treating risk factors for heart disease can also affect the risk of disease to other major organs.

On a regular basis, the ACC and AHA update their guidelines based on continued research and practice. Their goal is always to address the question of what the most important things are that need to be treated or controlled in order to stave off heart disease.

The ACC/AHA 2013 *Guidelines on the Assessment of Cardiovascular Risk* have been put into an algorithm called the CV Risk Calculator (cvriskcalculator.com). The site is accessible to all to calculate their risk using their own recent test result numbers. The algorithm analyzes the following data points: a person's age, gender, race, total cholesterol, HDL cholesterol, systolic and diastolic blood pressure, and whether that person is being treated for high blood pressure, has diabetes, or is a smoker. Simply entering a person's data into the calculator allows the algorithm to compute the chances of that person having a heart attack in the next ten years.

This simple calculation can support a doctor's suggestions: "Hey, you're at higher risk. Maybe you should watch what you eat by doing XYZ," or "Maybe we should adjust your cholesterol medication or get your blood pressure under better control." Granted there are some factors such as age, gender, and race that remain unalterable. But doctors and patients together can do something about the other factors such as cholesterol, blood pressure, diabetes, and smoking. A patient can stop smoking, can take medicine, and can make behavioral changes to help control blood pressure, diabetes, and cholesterol.

Knowing these risk factors for heart disease allows doctors to plan accordingly and can be an eye-opening motivator for patients. It may not seem as if treatment for high blood pressure or for diabetes is necessarily curative, but the ultimate goal in treating these is to decrease the risk for heart attack, stroke, and other cardiovascular diseases.

The Predictive Capacity of AI

As you might imagine, quite a lot of research goes into determining risk factors. The ACC and AHA assemble a panel of experts who comb the research and who have deep knowledge of the disease processes. They review all current medical knowledge in order to determine or reassess primary risk factors. In a sense, the identification of these factors is the ultimate scientific statement. All physicians rely on it because there's no getting any more thorough than that.

Or is there?

What's important to consider here is that the ACC/AHA guidelines *are the product of already completed research.* We know that it takes a long time for research to get to a point where it can be used in practice. For example, the current ACC guidelines account for years of research conducted by hundreds of researchers working all over the world, running clinical trials and other studies, writing papers, and coming up with hypotheses, recommendations, and solutions. Then, teams of experts joined as a work group, in which thousands of hours were committed to analyzing all of these efforts in order to put together a comprehensive list of risk factors based on all the research that has been completed to date.

Now imagine how AI would address this same project. AI essentially starts out with no need for "research" in the traditional sense. If given access to the EHR data for hundreds of thousands of people (both living and dead), would it be able to offer more accurate and more thorough predictive capacity than a panel of human doctors?

Stephen Weng, an epidemiologist at the University of Nottingham in the United Kingdom, conducted a study in an attempt to answer this question.[14] Weng's specific question was straightforward: Can machine learning improve cardiovascular risk prediction simply by using routine clinical data? Weng and his team compared four different machine learning algorithms. For those of you who are interested, those four algorithm types are called random forest, logistic regression, gradient boosting machine, and neural networks, and they are different methodologies for constructing computer algorithms. In Weng's study, the machines, essentially, taught themselves what they needed to know by reviewing and analyzing data from over 375,000 individuals' EHR records, looking for patterns of association with cardiovascular disease. The machines could also "see" more data points than were accounted for by the humans guiding the study.

The result of Weng's investigation? All four algorithms were more

---

14   S. Weng et al., "Can Machine-Learning Improve Cardiovascular Risk Prediction Using Routine Clinical Data?" PLoS ONE 12, no. 4 (April 4, 2017), https://doi.org/10.1371/journal.pone.0174944.

successful predictors than the ACC/AHA guidelines. Not only that, but the best among the algorithms accurately predicted 7.6 percent more events than the ACC/AHA guidelines and arrived at fewer false alarms. That might seem like a relatively small percentage, but in the study (which encompassed a period of time that had already passed), it amounted to an additional 355 patients who could have been treated and whose lives could have been saved or extended had they known they were at risk. That's 355 lives that were at risk and 355 more heart attacks and more deaths that could have been prevented.

AI Successes

Weng's study drew the following conclusions:

1. Any of these four algorithms that the machines used were better predictors of heart attacks than the method offered by the ACC/AHA guidelines. But there are even more insights that we can draw from Weng's study.

2. AI is much faster than human calculation. A team of expert doctors spends months poring over the data from clinical trials and other studies. By comparison, the machine goes *zoot*—maybe it completed its calculation in mere minutes— and generates more accurate results.

3. The ACC/AHA guidelines currently use eight variables or data points. By analyzing patient medical record data, the AI machines were able to review a lot more than eight variables to arrive at their results. In fact, the machines tested *thirty* variables in all.

4. AI was therefore able to discover more patterns of association and more risk factors from having considered more data points. Some of the very interesting risk factors that came to light in the AI study were arthritis, severe mental illness, the use of antipsychotic drugs, and the use of oral corticosteroids. The machines could also make some interesting associations between the likelihood of disease and patients' socioeconomic circumstances. For example, AI looked at the Townsend Deprivation Index, which measures material deprivation by examining the health effects of unemployment, household overcrowding, and the absence of car ownership and/or home ownership.

5. The predictive capacity of the machines suggests that if AI had access to even more data points, there may be even more variables *that we don't yet know of* that could help in predicting heart disease.

6. AI has the capacity to distinguish among populations. Whereas the ACC/AHA guidelines are basically the absolute standard for everybody in the world, there may be some odd risk factors that are not significant in certain populations but are very significant in others. For example, living in a particular geographical area might put someone at higher risk, or belonging to a particular ethnic community might act as a protective factor against certain widely recognized risk factors. The machine would be able to pick up those population-level details faster and more accurately than any human intuition, or even any clinical trial, could claim to do.

7. This conclusion is much like the previous one in terms of AI's capacity to enhance microlevel distinctions: using AI allows

us to see *variance* among risk factors. Take, for example, the risk factor of diabetes. So as far as we know now, a patient who has diabetes will always have diabetes, in the sense that diabetes is rarely curable. In general, once diagnosed, diabetes will be there for the rest of a patient's life. But we haven't yet asked whether treating the disease aggressively and managing the patient's blood sugar level within a very narrow "normal" range could lower the risk of cardiovascular disease. In other words, does it matter if the patient has diabetes or not, as long as that disease is being treated well and aggressively controlled?

Obviously, the ACC guidelines do not take this last scenario into account. But a machine can track data in both the short and long term and determine which of the risk factors is most significant—for a population, *or even for an individual.*

Let's conduct a comparison using the Weng study once again. The ACC/AHA guidelines indicate that even though men and women are different, age seems to be the most significant risk factor, and it's a factor we can't control. But of the controllable factors, we might ask questions such as whether controlling total cholesterol is better than controlling or stopping smoking. According to the guidelines, the answer is likely to be yes. So, doctor and patient might work on controlling cholesterol first because that's a bigger risk factor. Smoking comes next in the lineup.

ACC/AHA Algorithm		Machine-learning Algorithms			
Men	**Women**	**ML: Logistic Regression**	**ML: Random Forest**	**ML: Gradient Boosting Machines**	**ML: Neural Networks**
Age	Age	Ethnicity	Age	Age	Atrial Fibrillation
Total Cholesterol	HDL Cholesterol	Age	Gender	Gender	Ethnicity
HDL Cholesterol	Total Cholesterol	SES: Townsend Deprivation Index	Ethnicity	Ethnicity	Oral Corticosteroid Prescribed
Smoking	Smoking	Gender	Smoking	Smoking	Age
Age x Total Cholesterol	Age x *HDL Cholesterol*	*Smoking*	*HDL cholesterol*	*HDL cholesterol*	Severe Mental Illness
Treated Systolic Blood Pressure	Age x Total Cholesterol	Atrial Fibrillation	HbA1c	Triglycerides	SES: Townsend Deprivation Index
Age x Smoking	Treated Systolic Blood Pressure	Chronic Kidney Disease	Triglycerides	Total Cholesterol	Chronic Kidney Disease
Age x *HDL Cholesterol*	Untreated Systolic Blood Pressure	Rheumatoid Arthritis	SES: Townsend Deprivation Index	HbA1c	*BMI Missing*
Untreated Systolic Blood Pressure	Age x Smoking	Family history of premature CHD	BMI	Systolic Blood Pressure	Smoking
Diabetes	Diabetes	COPD	Total Cholesterol	SES: Townsend Deprivation Index	Gender

Table 1. Italics: Protective Factors. Source: Can machine-learning improve cardiovascular risk prediction using routine clinical data? PLOS ONE. https://doi.org/10.1371/journal.pone.0174944.t003.

Now, when we look at the Weng study, very different risk factors are prioritized. Ethnicity seems to be the number-one risk factor in the logistic regression model, followed by age. In the neural networks algorithm, the most significant risk is atrial fibrillation, something that ACC/AHA guidelines don't even look at! Atrial fibrillation shows up pretty high in the list of top factors identified in the logistic regression model as well. Its appearance in both models suggests that we should be paying closer attention to this factor than we do now.

Smoking, unsurprisingly, clearly plays a significant role, according to all of the algorithms. But what other previously unnoticed factors play a significant role, according to AI? Well, to give an example, oral corticosteroids, which are prescribed for asthma and some immune diseases, are a big contributor to risk in the AI study, as is severe mental illness.

One especially noteworthy risk factor, absent from the ACC/AHA guidelines but ranked fairly highly by all four algorithms, is the Townsend Deprivation Index, a measure, as I mentioned, of socioeconomic status. The algorithms support a conclusion that is only now gaining some attention in the way we think about prevention: education and other socioeconomic conditions powerfully affect health risk factors.

While the ACC/AHA models rank diabetes as the tenth most important risk factor, diabetes doesn't show up at all as a top risk factor in the AI study. On the other hand, HbA1c, a test of a patient's blood sugar over the course of months and used to monitor diabetes, *does* show up as a significant risk factor. So, your blood sugar is a more significant predictor of the risk of heart problems than the diagnosis of diabetes itself. In other words, to begin answering the question we asked about diabetes earlier in the chapter, simply having diabetes may not be as significant as the ACC/AHA guidelines seem to indicate. It is how well diabetes is controlled or not controlled that matters.

Those are just some of the interesting things we can draw from this one AI study that aren't also considered in the ACC guidelines. Not only can AI drill down and provide more accurate predictions but AI can also make more accurate predictions much faster than any human or team of humans.

One other extraordinary thing that AI can do is keep track of real-time changes. This is perhaps number eight in our running list of benefits that AI could bring to clinical practice.

Let's take a moment to explore this possibility. Say you have a population in Northern California for which you've been providing aggressive treatment and closely following patient response. Now, we know that risk factors change over time. If you checked the measurement today rather than in six months or one year, you might see a change in factors. Maybe the top ten risk factors will not be exactly the same. If this happens, your priorities might change, too, so far as controlling the risks are concerned.

It would be great to conduct this assessment often so that as the risks change within a given population, a physician's priorities in treating risk factors for disease within that population can change accordingly. The advantage of having a machine learning system in place to assist with clinical practice is that doctors can take far more frequent snapshots of the population they are treating. Changes can be made more regularly, more in line with the timing of actual changes in patient conditions. It's also likely that taking these more frequent snapshots provides not only a more accurate picture of disease processes but is also less costly.

In this chapter, we've been considering the value of AI disease prediction *in a population*, whether that's within a particular geographic region or even within a particular clinical practice. But point number eight hints at the capacity for AI to recognize and analyze the very specific functions and needs *of individual patients*. For now, it's worth remembering that the way medicine works is to take what we know about human beings in general and then determine how best to apply that knowledge in an individual case. And individuals, as we know, can have a host of very specific issues and quirks that do not reflect the state of "knowledge in general." Being attentive to the particularities of each patient is a tremendously daunting task. And that makes it very challenging to find the right balance between the general rule and the particular case to be able successfully to treat and prevent disease.

It's to the matter of AI's contributions to precision *in diagnosis* that I will turn in the next chapter, as we continue to explore the revolutionary potentials that machine learning can have in finding exactly what works for each and every patient.

CHAPTER 4

Diagnosis:
The Background

I n the story of the elephant and the five blind men, five blind men were assigned the task of describing an elephant. There was one problem: they had never come across an elephant before. They were led to an elephant, which they started touching. The first man touched the trunk and declared that the elephant was a large snake. Another man felt the ear and said that the elephant was a large fan. Yet another man felt the tail of the animal and said it was a rope. The fourth man touched a tusk and said the elephant was a spear. The last man felt the side of the elephant and said it was a wall. None of the blind men got the full picture of the elephant.

Sometimes the diagnostic process is complex. We may be seeing short windows of a patient's history and symptoms, and we are not sure how the pieces fit together as a whole. This may be because the patients only visit the doctor sporadically, or because various specialists treat only individual aspects of the disease, or because there are gaps in our knowledge of how the disease develops and ends. In other words, the diagnosis and treatment processes don't match the specifics of the illness they're intended to uncover or confirm. What happens instead is that those processes can far exceed or even be irrelevant to what doctors most need to know. Let me explain.

Most of us are aware that a doctor needs to run tests in order to be able to diagnose a condition. What may not be so obvious to some of us is that reimbursement is based on the tests run, diagnosis made, or treatment given. The formula is simple: the more severe the diagnosis, the higher the reimbursement. In other words, physicians need a diagnosis in order to treat a condition, but they also need it for reimbursement and to justify paying for the tests and the treatments that follow. Sometimes other tests are ordered to rule out certain diagnoses, as a way of decreasing the chances of missing something. Other times, diagnostic tests are done to satisfy a regulatory requirement. So, although a diagnosis serves the purpose of treating the patient, sometimes it is done to increase reimbursement, to protect the physician in case of a law suit, or to satisfy a regulatory requirement. None of the above reasons may actually help the patient. This is how the utilization and cost of testing keeps increasing, and this process ultimately leads to overdiagnosis and overtreatment.

Wastefulness is spread across current diagnostic practices. Part of the reason for this wastefulness is that our practices follow a set formula that, essentially, encourages unnecessary testing.

Right now, the system works by subjecting every patient who comes in with a particular problem or complaint to a set of routine steps predetermined and agreed upon by the medical community. Even though there may be instances in which running a whole lot of tests can seem reassuring both to patients and, especially, to worried family members, the process may not be tailored to the individual patient. A set of due diligence diagnostic procedures take effect whenever a patient manifests a specific symptom or set of symptoms. Granted, this makes sense insofar as health care professionals rely on the existence of routine tests that help determine what's going on with any individual patient. Diseases, injuries, conditions—they tend to manifest themselves in relatively similar ways in all individuals. However, this same sense-making process gives rise to a lot of waste. It is a process that could really be improved upon.

Say a patient comes to the emergency room (ER), complaining of chest pain. There are guidelines to which we currently refer when determining what could be the cause of that pain and they take physician and patients through a set series of steps. It's a one-size-fits-all approach. Everybody who comes in with that complaint gets the same battery of tests in basically the same order. That's because human judgments about probability are at stake, and these tests help doctors make judgments about patients' potential for heart damage or disease.

Now let's drill down a bit on this issue of testing. There are two parameters that we have to keep in mind. One concerns the characteristics of the test. Each test has two different characteristics: sensitivity and specificity. Every test result has four possibilities: true positives, true negatives, false positives, and false negatives. Essentially, sensitivity is a measure of true positives or true positive rate, which means that in the case of a test with high sensitivity, you will have fewer false negatives. Specificity is a measure of true negatives or true negative rate. A test with high specificity will have fewer false negatives. Ideally a test should have 100 percent sensitivity and 100 percent specificity, but this is never the case in the real world—which is to say, in actual practice.

The second parameter is the characteristic of the population being tested or the population the individual is coming from. In addition to sensitivity and specificity, the utility of a test is based on the prevalence of disease or of the factor being tested for. There are two measures that we use for this. They are called positive predictive value and negative predictive value. Positive predictive value refers to the proportion of people who have the disease when the test is positive. Remember that just because a test is positive, it does not necessarily mean that the person has the disease, because sometimes the test can be falsely positive. So, also, the negative predictive value is the proportion of people *not* having a disease when the test is negative. In other words, the same test performs differently in two populations based on the prevalence of the disease in each population.

Each test is going to have a certain sensitivity and specificity. And then there is the prevalence of the disease in the population. The determination of which test to use depends on the purpose of testing, whether one is trying to rule in a disease or rule out a disease and the prevalence of the disease in the population. In each case, doctors are questioning the chances of a person having the disease for which they are testing. A low prevalence of the disease might favor the use of a test with high sensitivity. But if the chances of having the disease are high, a different test with high specificity might be used. Not understanding or using this knowledge leads to a lot of unnecessary testing, including preventable downstream testing. It leads, as well, to missing a diagnosis or to over diagnosing.

Let's take breast cancer as our example here, and let's assume that there is a 2 percent prevalence of breast cancer in the population, which means 2 in every 100 women have breast cancer. If we want to test all 100 women, we would pick a test that has a high true positive rate or one with high sensitivity. We want to have a low false negative rate, so we use a high-sensitivity test, in this case, a mammogram or x-ray of the breasts that reveals suspicious areas for cancer. But the test does not necessarily have to be specific—which means it may detect some false positives—but it will not miss patients who are true positives. Now say we run this test on 100 women, and the test picks up five people as positive. We need to test these five people with a high-specificity test and high true negatives. This next test could be a biopsy, where a sample of the tissue is taken from the breast and tested for cancer cells under a microscope. This test will tell us with a high degree of certainty which three women do not have breast cancer and which two do. So, we used a highly specific test to screen 100 women and a highly sensitive test to rule out a diagnosis in the smaller group of five women. Now consider what would happen if we switched the order of the tests. The biopsy, other than being expensive, inconvenient, labor intensive, painful, and difficult to do if a detectable lump is not present, would have missed too many patients who are actually starting to develop a tumor. If we were to use the mammogram as a second test, it would pick up too many false positives and would put patients through unnecessary treatments such as surgery. Also note that the positive predictive value and negative predictive value are different for these two populations of 100 women and 5 women because the prevalence of the disease is different.

		DISEASE				
		+	(-)	Total		
TEST	+	2	3	5	PPV	0.40
	(-)	0	95	95	NPV	1.00
	Total	2	98	100		
		SNS	SPC			
		1.00	0.97			

Table 2. A 2 x 2 table showing the characteristics of a screening test. SNS: Sensitivity; SPC: Specificity; PPV: Positive Predictive Value; NPV: Negative Predictive Value.

As shown in Table 2, I took a very simple example to demonstrate the principles of testing. Imagine that, in medicine, there are very complex situations, myriads of tests with varying degrees of sensitivity and specificity, and conditions with a wide range of prevalence in a wide variety of populations. We can see how quickly the matter of testing and diagnosing becomes extremely complicated.

If we have a way for the machine to determine and calculate all these variables, it should be able to suggest ways that we could drastically cut down on waste and improve diagnostic accuracy. This would be even more the case if we were able to tailor the diagnostic procedures to the individual patient, even just to some degree. The capacity of AI to help predetermine which tests would fit for a particular patient in a particular population can dramatically reduce our chances both of missing a diagnosis and of treating people for diseases they do not actually have.

The Immense Value of Machine Accuracy

Let's think about how machine diagnosis compares to human doctor diagnosis. Right away, on the human side, we know we're using the current method of evaluating a patient that I mentioned earlier in this chapter, which is to follow a set list of items in the charting or documentation system. When examining the heart, for example, doctors look for things such as murmurs, irregular beats, the rate, and the rhythm. Those are the things we know to begin with in order to identify any irregularities. The characteristics that doctors look for in arriving at a particular diagnosis are regulated by the need to satisfactorily run through the set diagnostic steps that reflect longstanding habits and current knowledge.

AI, however, should be able to tell us which specific test or finding we should focus on for a particular patient, getting us to the right answer faster, with more precision, and without unnecessary effort. In other words, AI gives us *more predictive information* about what next steps to take in each particular case, and because of that, AI should be able to give us a better prediction of pretest probability. *Before any test is run on a patient*, we would already have a firm sense of the probability of this particular patient having the disease. Knowing the pretest probability, we can then tell which test is the better one for this specific person who shows potential for having this specific condition.

Let's return to the example of a patient complaining of chest pain, and this time, let's say that patient goes to the ER. That's actually a very regular occurrence. Chest pain is one of the top three complaints seen in emergency rooms; of one hundred patients who go to the emergency room, roughly ten of them complain of chest pain. The standard procedure is to give each patient who comes in with chest pain an EKG, blood tests, a short stay for observation, a treadmill test, and so on. If we had an AI system that could take the patient's current data, analyze it in relation to the patient's ongoing and past data, compare it with others who have gone through the same process, and predict the probability of this patient having a heart attack in the next seven days, thirty days, one year, five years, and so on—which, given enough data, an AI system can do—we may not have to do all of these tests in the ER. We could have a much stronger sense of which tests would be most useful for each specific patient. AI could drastically cut down on the costs for hospital admissions, work-ups, tests, procedures, and doctor time, all while decreasing anxiety for the patient and getting that person home faster.

In the United States, an effort is already underway to reduce unnecessary diagnostics. It should not be a surprise to learn that this effort tends to be part of a larger push to recognize the value-based care model that we discussed in chapter 2 and it has been focused, especially, on diagnostic imaging. Diagnostic imaging is an important area, not only because it is expensive but also because it has the potential for doing harm to patients through radiation exposure. Radiation to the body increases the risk of cancer in the longer term, though its deleterious effects may not be seen in the shorter term. Were we to have a system that could track long-term outcomes, it could guide physicians by calculating the risk associated with undergoing an imaging test versus the benefit of finding a treatable problem.

I want to draw attention to the significance of AI when it comes to reading images. When you think about it, the nice thing about imaging is that it's very, very straightforward. So far, some of the great advances in AI have been made in the area of imaging, because machines are really good at reading images, picking up differences between images, and identifying what the images are showing. AI can break an image down into tiny pixels and look for arrangements or pixel patterns. Any image can be analyzed in terms of its different color or light values—for example, a shade of color or a shade of darkness. That's completely measurable by AI. The machine can come to "see" a disease or condition at a very granular level and then compare the patterns it identifies with previous knowledge it has gained from looking at similar patterns in thousands of similar images. That is why diagnostic imaging is one of the areas of medicine where AI has been very useful already. We could say that diagnostic imaging is an early adopter of AI, or at least, we could say that AI should be used across the board for reading images and pointing out where doctors should focus their attention.

Comparing AI to Humans

Studies have already looked into the differences between physicians' readings of images and AI readings of images in order to measure and compare the accuracy of each. In one study conducted by researchers at Stanford, a neural network developed the ability to read chest x-rays in order to detect pneumonia.[15] The network did a better job identifying the disease than a test group of radiologists. The focus on pneumonia was an important part of the study because early diagnosis of that disease is critical to preventing further complications and death. Not only did the neural network do a better job with pneumonia detection, but it was better at finding over a dozen other diseases, too. In this study, the interesting thing was not simply to see if the machine could best the practicing radiologists but also to show that the success of the machine could especially help patients in areas of the world where there are shortages of radiologists to interpret x-rays. In other words, one of the tremendous untapped benefits of AI is that it could help more people get the diagnostic information they need.

Another study along these same lines showed the use of AI to crowdsource medical knowledge from doctors across seventy countries.[16] This is another way in which AI could help transmit the advice of specialists to general practitioners in a timely and cost-effective way. Machine algorithms have also had greater success than human experts at identifying heart arrhythmias, spotting cancerous skin

---

15 P. Rajpurkar et al., "CheXNet: Radiologist-Level Pneumonia Detection on Chest X-Rays with Deep Learning," arXiv (electronic archive), December 2017, Cornell University Libraries, https://arxiv.org/pdf/1711.05225.pdf.

16 Jeremy Hsu, "Can a Crowdsourced AI Medical Diagnosis App Outperform Your Doctor?" *Scientific American*, August 11, 2017, https://www.scientificamerican.com/article/can-a-crowdsourced-ai-medical-diagnosis-app-outperform-your-doctor.

lesions, screening for diabetic retinopathy, and even differentiating cancer cells from normal cells.[17]

It's not hard to understand why AI imaging diagnostics are more *accurate* than the human eye, and when you add the factor of human fatigue, AI also seems a more *reliable* measuring tool. Looking at x-rays or pathology slides all day is very tedious and painful. It's true that looking at more images gives a doctor more experience and success. That's why more experienced pathologists and more experienced radiologists do a better job of identifying abnormalities. But as doctors look at more and more x-rays in a day, serious fatigue can set in, which can decrease accuracy because fatigue reduces the power of perception. The considerable amount of time it takes to read x-rays is another disadvantage. Reading a chest x-ray requires examining each structure, each layer, each shadow. Plus, human brains need breaks when working hard. We humans cannot work continuously. Finally, we can be distracted. Our brains multitask. A human brain might not just be reading x-rays; it might also be thinking about what to cook for dinner, or how to proceed with a research project, or when to schedule a meeting with the boss.

And other human factors get in the way. Doctors occasionally simply miss some things, even very obvious things, because the human brain is not 100 percent accurate in its abilities to detect. That's the stress of practicing medicine: "Oh my gosh, did I miss something?" There is a miss rate that is always there; it cannot be zero. However good physicians may be, their error rate will never be zero.

Machines, on the other hand, have proven to be very good at

---

17   A. Esteva et al., "Dermatologist-Level Classification of Skin Cancer with Deep Neural Networks," *Nature* 542, no. 7639 (February 2, 2017): 115–118, https://doi.org/10.1038/nature21056; R. Gargeya and T. Leng, "Automated Identification of Diabetic Retinopathy Using Deep Learning," *Ophthalmology* 124, no. 7 (July 2017): 962-969, https://doi.org/10.1016/j.ophtha.2017.02.008.

recognizing patterns and details. And with machine learning, more is actually better: the more a machine sees, the better it gets at identifying; each new image is a pure opportunity for learning. Unlike humans, who have to train new generations of doctors to be able to carry on their work, machine learning can be easily replicated. The experience and the knowledge of one machine can be transferred to others *without anything being lost in the process.* The copy of the machine is as good as the original. Machines don't suffer fatigue as human beings do. And machine analysis is very fast. As a machine gets trained and has extra computing power added to it, it becomes faster at recognizing patterns and details. Finally, machine reading is more easily scalable, especially in terms of speed and volume. In human practice, the number of pictures that can be read depends on the number of radiologists or pathologists on staff, whereas a single machine can continue to read, day and night, all the while increasing accuracy.

Granted, all of these benefits depend on a machine *being given enough data.* And that could become a bit of a sticking point, because we only collect data we already believe is going to be useful. Using AI in the way I am suggesting would mean that we would always have to ask ourselves whether other important data remain uncollected. This could be tricky since, on the one hand, we want to reduce the data we collect to only the necessary data, but on the other hand, we do not know with any certainty which data are going to prove valuable for making certain diagnoses.

It is best to think about using AI in medicine as a kind of assistive partnership between machines and health care professionals. There may be factors relevant to diagnostic processes that humans do not yet know they need to find out about. As we pursue the incorporation of AI into clinical practice, we will have to take great care not to leave out of our data collection items that could come to be important factors. AI may be able to give us the hints or suggestions we need to determine which bits of information may be the truly useful to collect from patients. Inversely, it can also decrease physicians' workloads by identifying irrelevant data points that have been traditionally collected through health records. There may also be methods of conducting lab tests and analyzing the results that humans have not yet discovered. There may even be modes of analysis that the human brain will never be able to devise.

One thing, though, is clear: The success of AI shows us that we are at a turning point in the way we learn about and make sense of the human body and the practice of medicine.

Benefits to All Three Stakeholder Groups

The diagnostic capacity of AI is beneficial to all three of our stakeholders: doctors, health care companies, and patients.

Doctors can have some of their cognitive workload or problem-solving burden offset by AI which, as an assistive technology, would help doctors diagnose more rapidly and more accurately. With the assistance of AI, doctors can become even better at what they do and can use their freed cognitive space for other functions such as more advanced thinking and closer interaction with patients. Each advance in technology, or the emergence of an entirely new technology, has helped physicians become better at what they do. For example, the invention of the stethoscope greatly improved a physician's ability to hear a patient's heart and breathing as opposed to putting an ear to the patient's chest. With each new technology, physicians' work becomes a bit easier and more efficient.

Companies, for which the costs of care are paramount, would likely reap the benefit of seeing particular costs decreased. The expenses associated with diagnostic error—when physicians fail to detect a patient's disease or mistakenly diagnose and treat a disease the patient actually doesn't have—increase the bad outcomes. Minimally, these two sources of increased costs could be decreased with the help of AI.

AI clearly benefits patients through a more accurate and quicker diagnosis. Speed is key: when patients don't have to wait for various tests or go through a treatment trial and error process, they discover more quickly what's ailing them. Lowering the likelihood of patients having to go through unnecessary treatment or unnecessary tests should improve their overall experience, and patients who do have a high likelihood of a particular diagnosis will get aggressive treatment more quickly.

At the start of this chapter, we considered the growing wastefulness of diagnostic testing in current health care practice. I hope by now it is clear that an AI-centric approach to diagnostic processes could cut that waste significantly. In particular, *AI can make diagnosis more accurate, less time consuming, and ultimately, less costly.* I'd argue that nearly every new medical technology has led to improvements in these three areas. AI is no different, in this sense, from past technological achievements in medicine.

A Word on Physicians' Resistance

Before we move on to a closer look at two examples of AI's use in diagnostics, I want to address, head-on and just briefly for now, the idea that AI can make a physician's job easier. Many doctors hear about the great success of new medical technologies, especially ones that can take on some of their tasks and improve upon their performance, and they worry that technology will, ultimately, make their jobs obsolete. Will AI decrease the number of physicians that are needed to do the same job? Maybe it will. Will it take away physicians' jobs? No, because there are so many other things that physicians need to do and, currently, don't have enough time to do. Might AI make certain specializations in medicine less enticing to new medical students? Maybe. But that might only mean that even newer areas of specialization will arise, or that specialization in medicine will become less and less the norm and a different way of thinking about practicing medicine will emerge. Typically, when new technologies have come into the picture, physicians have expanded their expertise in other areas. For example, when new catheter-guided procedures became popular, cardiologists and radiologists became interventionalists. Instead of reading x-rays and CT scans, radiologists started conducting procedures using imaging guidance. And cardiologists, who were mostly treating patients with medications, went on to become invasive cardiologists and started performing angioplasties. New technologies offer new opportunities to grow a skill set and specialize. I believe that AI will be no different; it will open up many doors for physicians in and beyond their respective specialties.

Any fearful anticipation of AI's effects on the practice of medicine is simply fear of the unknown. Depending on how we decide to make best use of the technology, AI is likely to replace the less advanced functions of a physician's job. It can empower a radiologist to perform more focused work by identifying areas of high priority for review, or by helping eliminate from review x-rays that read as normal, or by reading x-rays when radiologists are unavailable. In any case, AI is likely to be best utilized as an assistive technology that can free doctors to focus their efforts on the things that humans are better at than machines, such as consulting on differential diagnoses. There will always be the human side of a physician's job that a machine cannot do in the same way, or with the same benefit, or even, quite frankly, at all.

That said, I want to acknowledge that assistive technologies do sometimes lead to radical changes to the way physicians work, and AI is very likely to do that in the future, for diagnostic procedures in particular. But the question we should be asking in response to advances in AI is not whether we should use AI as a diagnostic tool in clinical practice but, rather, how we can use this new technology to find disease and save lives, how soon physicians can learn and transition to working with these new technologies, and how we can help make that transition a positive and successful experience for everyone involved. After all, the physicians who are able to adapt to working with the newer technologies are the ones who will move their careers and their practices forward.

CHAPTER 5

Diagnosis: The Application

I n reviewing the use of AI as a diagnostic tool, I've pointed out two different areas of use. One is the ability of machines to teach themselves to read and analyze images. In this chapter, I want to look closely at another example that returns to a point we have already spent some time thinking about in earlier chapters: the ability of machines to teach themselves to scan and analyze large amounts of data. Let's dig into a specific example of that now.

Diagnosing Sepsis

Let's consider another emergency room example: Paramedics bring to the emergency room a sixty-eight-year-old woman with generalized weakness. She lives alone at her home and has not been able to get up to prepare her meals for the last twenty-four hours. She is alert and oriented but appears weak. Her vital signs are normal. She has no fever. She gets blood tests, urine tests and x-rays done in the emergency care unit, and these are all normal except for her chest x-ray, which shows a patchy shadow in her right lung. She is diagnosed with pneumonia, started on antibiotics, and admitted to the medical ward. Later that evening, when the nurse comes to check her vital signs, she is altered mentally and her blood pressure has dropped. She is diagnosed with septic shock and is transferred to the intensive care unit (ICU) for aggressive treatment and close monitoring.

Sepsis is a serious clinical condition associated with high mortality rates in hospitalized patients. Sepsis presents as the classic fever and infection scenario. The infection can be anywhere in the body. When septic, the whole body reacts and, eventually, the compensatory mechanisms will fail, the blood pressure starts to fall, and the body goes into shock. Septic shock carries a pretty high mortality rate of 25–30 percent if not recognized early, and 10–12 percent if recognized early.[18]

The hospitalization of patients with sepsis lasts much longer and is more expensive than that of the average hospital patient. If sepsis is diagnosed early and treated aggressively with intravenous fluids and intravenous antibiotics, patient outcomes are more favorable. The sooner the diagnosis is made, and the sooner the treatment is started, the better the outcomes. The trouble with diagnosing sepsis is this: it is hard to detect early using traditional methods, and once its onset has occurred, it is extremely destructive, extremely quickly.

Sepsis presents a diagnostic challenge: it responds well to treatment when diagnosed and treated early, but it is difficult to

---

18   For a quick reference point, see the Sepsis Alliance's *Sepsis Fact Sheet* (Adobe PDF) under Sepsis FAQ at https://www.sepsis.org/faq. For more detailed information, see Florian B. Mayr, Sachin Yende, and Derek C. Angus, "Epidemiology of Severe Sepsis," *Virulence* 5, no. 1 (January 1, 2014): 4–11, https://doi.org/10.4161/viru.27372.

diagnose early, and our current methods of predicting and diagnosing it are not particularly reliable.

Predicting and diagnosing sepsis involves looking at vital signs, laboratory data, and clinical observation. Vital signs are tracked by monitoring devices, but lab and clinical observation data *require a physician's suspicion of sepsis* to trigger any action. Once a physician suspects the condition, there are still delays, including the time it takes to order a lab test, complete the lab test, report the results, determine the treatment, and, finally, to order and deliver the treatment. This lag time is crucial: each hour the problem has not been recognized or addressed puts the patient in greater danger. In an ideal situation, we would require minimal data for diagnosis, and data would be routinely collected rather than reliant upon the physician coming into the room to observe the patient.

The Traditional Method of Diagnosis

As I've already noted, we currently diagnose sepsis by looking at symptoms and a lab test. The symptoms are fever, fast heartbeat, fast breathing, high temperature or low temperature, and, sometimes, low blood pressure. These are called systemic inflammatory response syndrome (SIRS) criteria. Physicians look at the constellation of all of these symptoms along with a blood test for serum lactate or lactic acid. Severe sepsis is present if the lactic acid is above a certain level. If the lactic acid level is high and the blood pressure is low, you have a case of septic shock. Both are part of the spectrum of the same disease.

Additionally, as I've noted, the mainstay of the treatment is antibiotics and the fast delivery of quite a lot of IV fluids. There are other medications and treatments available after the initial course of antibiotics and fluids. When sepsis is recognized early, it can be treated early, in which case, treatment is fairly effective. Mortality rates can be dropped by half or more when treatment is given early and fast. Mortality goes up with any delays.

According to the current diagnostic model, however, *patients are already septic before they are formally determined to be so.* Add to this fact all the delays that happen once a sepsis diagnosis is made. Frankly, even after the doctor gets to the point of placing the order for treatment, it's still the case that the pharmacy has to mix the antibiotic and send it to the ward, and the nurse has to prepare it, start an intravenous line, and hang it. At a minimum, it takes an hour or two for that whole part of the process to happen. And that's just to get the antibiotic portion of the treatment started.

Having recognized that the current science is truly insufficient in this area, a team of researchers with which I'm involved decided to ask whether it is possible to predict or diagnose sepsis in hospitalized patients earlier than we do now.

The AI Method of Diagnosis

We applied machine learning techniques to address this challenging question and developed algorithms that can use routine vital sign data to predict sepsis *several hours before its onset.* Machines alert physicians to the increasing possibility of sepsis developing in a patient. This allows physicians to order confirmatory tests and start treatment sooner so that a patient's condition does not become critical.

Here's what we did:[19]

In the ICU, a variety of continuously collected data can be used to track trends in the patients' status and make predictions about their stability. Clinical decision support systems (CDSSs) are the tools health care providers use to make these predictions and evaluate the severity of a patient's condition. But the CDSSs currently in use offer less than optimal results. In fact, they can fail to identify nearly 60 percent of unstable patients.

Research already has shown that certain AI tools and machine learning techniques using this EHR data can help predict patient instability and mortality and in forecasting other patient outcomes. Knowing this led us to ask more specifically whether EHR data alone can predict who will become septic. Our methodology looked at heart rate and blood pressure, and at a few of the other criteria used to identify sepsis.

What we found was that subtle changes in vital signs were enough to predict the onset of sepsis. Measuring vital signs enabled the machines to predict sepsis four, eight, twelve, and even twenty-four hours before its onset.

Instead of having to wait until after the completion of a blood test for sepsis to be diagnosed, our tool was able to predict sepsis and septic shock in the ICU before onset, allowing physicians to take preventative measures on behalf of their patients. In other words, our tool predicted sepsis before patients actually had sepsis, as currently defined.

To develop the tool, we took a large database of about forty thousand patients with all their vital signs—heart rate, respiratory rate, systolic and diastolic blood pressure, temperature, and pulse oximetry—and their medical history. Using those numbers, we

---

19   T Desautels et al., "Prediction of Sepsis in the Intensive Care Unit With Minimal Electronic Health Record Data: A Machine Learning Approach," *JMIR Med Inform* 4, no. 3 (September 2016), https://doi.org/10.2196/medinform.5909.

developed a model that can, if certain criteria are met, help us predict whether the patient will become septic.

You'll recall that besides looking at vital signs, the traditional scoring systems also take into consideration a potential laundry list of lab test results. These can be any number of tests including lactic acid, cell count, C-reactive protein, creatinine, and liver function tests. Yet a third contributor to the traditional system of diagnosis is the physician's physical examination of a patient's current condition.

Of these three routes to diagnosis, the vital signs are clearly the easiest to obtain because they are routinely taken. A doctor doesn't need to have a special order for vital sign data to be collected. Granted, these variables need not only to be taken but also to be reviewed or assessed frequently enough for trends to become visible. Especially in the case of sepsis, the precise time when the patient developed the condition must be identified. Beyond vital signs, you can see how the other two approaches to diagnosis—physician evaluation and lab testing—can delay the timely treatment of sepsis. When it comes to physical evaluation of a patient, there may be some factors that the physician might miss. Relevant information may not be mentioned in the medical record that the doctor sees when visiting a patient, *because that record does not include all the data from the EHR system.* It is even more likely that the physician may not be anticipating or suspecting sepsis in the first place and so may not even have looked for the physical signs of it. Given that lab tests are not ordered unless and until the physician suspects a problem, you can see how machine-tracking subtle changes in the patient improves upon the current model.

As our team discovered, the impending onset of sepsis can be picked up by vital signs alone. Tracking and analyzing vital signs, *in the absence of either lab tests or physician observation*, makes possible the detection of subtle changes that accompany the onset of sepsis.

The machine analysis, essentially, asks how these data points change, in relation to one another and tracked over time, when a patient is becoming septic. The analysis also asks which vital signs are becoming significant, which direction they are trending, what their magnitude is, and how the individual vital signs relate to one another.

Comparing Methodologies

There is an additional question to be posed here: Is it necessary to design or train algorithms each time they are put to use in new populations? For example, will the differences between the population in one area of the country and the population in a completely different area of the country require a fresh start, or can the machine's learning, say in a town in the northeastern United States, be applied to a town in the southwestern United States? One way to think about the significance of this question is by considering how traditional research methodologies work. Following traditional methods, a scientist begins with a problem, asks a research question, picks a population, or a sample of a population, to study, and then sets about the work of the conducting the study. The study results are, essentially, generalized to everyone. The implication of the traditional model tends to be: that what is found in a subset of a population will apply to the whole—and what is applicable to one population is applicable to another.

The AI methodology differs from the traditional method significantly on precisely this point. A researcher gathers data from the full population and then builds algorithms in order to test them. Those algorithms get reused, trained again in a new data set, and tested again. In a way, AI allows researchers to generate new knowledge with each iteration, as well as apply all the accumulated knowledge in addressing the most current cases. To reiterate: in the traditional model, small-scale research is applied with the expectation that it will work across the board. Furthermore, in the traditional model, there just aren't a lot of studies tracking implementation in and across various populations. With AI, however, learning can be continuous. As the process is ongoing and with each new population, the accuracy of the algorithm is finely tuned. The machine already knows some things, and it learns and adjusts to local variations as it is applied to them. Each algorithm is finely tuned to a specific population when it is being used for that population. In other words, in each use, the algorithm becomes smarter *for the population to which it is applied.*

What is unique here is that AI allows us to generate new knowledge about large populations and implement that knowledge nearly simultaneously. The effect for scientific research is that this process decreases, and could eliminate in the future, the time from bench (the research itself) to bedside (the implementation or application of the results of that research). Using AI, the time it takes to improve health outcomes is greatly condensed.

A second important point about its uniqueness is that AI can predict and diagnose successfully *in data-poor environments.* In the case of the sepsis study, all that was needed was to read a handful of vital signs with an understanding of how they change when a patient moves toward sepsis. Whether we can call this a tool for prediction or for early diagnosis, the end result is that early on, the physician receives a warning that a particular patient is headed toward a dangerous condition. The condition can be addressed before it is fully experienced by the patient, thereby giving the treatment an advantage against the illness.

That advantage is significant as it makes a difference in how quickly the patient responds to treatment and how long the patient must remain in the ICU and in the hospital. The AI methodology, insofar as it outperforms other more traditional measures, contributes both to saving patients from life-threatening situations and to saving health care costs overall.

The Precision of AI

In the next two chapters, we will focus on the use of AI to improve treatment. What I want to mention here, though, is something I think might already be obvious from the material we have covered so far. As AI models study more and more patients, they become more capable of determining which components of diagnosis are the most relevant ones and which components of complex treatments are more successful than others. Another quick sepsis example will, I hope, help solidify my point. The early 2000s saw the establishment of a detailed protocol called early goal directed therapy (EGDT).[20] The protocol consisted of several components, including the use of antibiotics, IV fluids, the measurement of pressures in the heart, and even blood transfusions. Initially, clinical trials showed positive results; use of this protocol seemed to save lives or keep people out of danger when they had sepsis. As time went on, however, other studies challenged these findings. There was the suggestion that not all parts of the protocol were necessary, or that the protocol itself was not particularly reliable. It took more than a decade for the medical community to determine that the protocol was actually unnecessary. Millions of dollars and years of implementing the protocol finally led to that determination.

---

20 Emanuel Rivers et al., "Early Goal-Directed Therapy in the Treatment of Severe Sepsis and Septic Shock," *N Engl J Med* 345, no. 19 (November 2001): 1368–77, https://doi.org/10.1056/NEJMoa010307.

But we have already seen the speed and the precision with which AI can teach itself to understand relationships among a tremendous number of data points. Now imagine the application of AI when it comes to medical treatment. As AI studies more and more patients, it can determine which components of any treatment plan are the ones that are most reliable, the ones that actually work for a given population, or, as we will see in what follows, for a given patient.

CHAPTER 6

Treatment: The Background

During the British rule in India, there was a major problem with cobras slithering around and creating havoc among the citizens. The government declared that the cobras were a menace to the population and ordered that they be killed. Citizens were offered monetary compensation for bringing dead cobras to the government office. Getting paid for turning in dead cobras quickly became an easy way to make money. Some citizens even became professional cobra catchers. Eventually, the citizens realized that catching cobras was becoming more and more difficult; the cobra population was actually dwindling. So, they came up with a plan. They would breed cobras so that they could kill them and make money. To their surprise, this had the effect of making the cobra problem worse!

In the same way that the citizens addressed the cobra problem by making it worse, our system of health care often addresses its own problems by exacerbating them. In the United States, every single year, billions of dollars are spent on unnecessary medical care. In part, this happens because of what I described in chapter 2 as the fee-for-service model of health care in which doctors are rewarded for ordering tests, doing procedures, and treating patients with medicines. But in the value-based system I'm advocating in this book, we could significantly reduce the amount of money spent on unnecessary treatments. That would also reduce the amount of monetary burden faced by patients who believe that they must pay for these treatments if they are to have a chance at health and life.

Saving money is a tremendously important piece of changing the system so as to better address patients' health needs. It is tied to rooting out unnecessary processes and to devising more accurate treatment practices.

Let's take treatments for hypertension as an example. The goal of treatment is to help patients take control of their blood pressure and set themselves up for better long-term outcomes such as decreased risk of heart attack or stroke. Now, different classes of drugs act on different pathways in the body to achieve the overall goal of decreasing blood pressure. Not only are there multiple classes of medication for hypertension, but there are even different types of medicines within the same class. When we begin a treatment for hypertension, we take into consideration all these differences, along with factors such as the age of the patient, the patient's race, and other medical conditions that the patient might be experiencing, and, ultimately, we look at the patient's response to the treatment to tell us if it is working appropriately.

A lot of people might expect there is one medication out there to treat each disease. But think about how we treat very common conditions such as depression. There are multiple drugs for the same condition. And the method we have for trying out a certain drug is to wait a few months and see if and how the patient responds to it. If the response is good, that's great. If it's not, then we switch to another drug and wait for another few weeks or months to see if the patient responds well, or doesn't. The more drugs that come into the market, the more difficult it becomes to find the right treatment, the right drugs, and the right protocol to address a given condition. The newest drug is not simply supposed to replace the one currently used; it is supposed to be an overall improvement. That may happen, but it is rare.

For many diseases, it is often the case that a combination of medicines, not just one medicine, may be necessary for symptom relief. But how do we select the combination? What should be the specific dosages of each of those medicines in that combination? Should a patient start taking the combination of medicines all at the same time, or should each medicine be tested serially? Those are very complicated issues that need to be understood, and our understanding often comes after the fact. In other words, we engage in a process of trial and error with medicines and patients to see what works. Of course, this does not mean that we assign medicines to patients willy-nilly. We still have to invest a lot of forethought and analysis in understanding what each drug does and how a set of drugs might work in combination with one another in a particular patient. But the very best indicator we have right now of *what will work* for a given patient is *what actually ends up working for that patient*.

Now, let's consider diseases that are very complicated and difficult to treat because the treatments themselves depend on a multitude of factors. For example, treating cancer is likely to involve chemotherapy, radiation therapy, surgery, and immunotherapy. Even just one of these areas—chemotherapy, for example—involves various combinations of medicines that could address a given type of cancer. This means that treatment protocols for the same cancer can vary greatly based on factors such as the development stage of the cancer, the primary organs affected, and the age and health status of the patient. In other words, cancer treatment itself is very complex: we have to generate a treatment protocol for a particular cancer with a particular histologic diagnosis at a particular stage and in a particular patient, because each of these variables affects the outcome.

A type of cancer treatment known as targeted therapy has begun to help us be more exact in treating a particular cancer. Targeted therapy treats certain cancer cells by blocking their ability to grow and spread. Targeted therapy is also the basis for what is called precision medicine, in which doctors attempt to understand how the genetic makeup of a given patient will have an effect on the medication selected. One example of this that has become widely known is the identification of the BRCA gene for breast cancer. We also see precision medicine at work in the treatment of some psychiatric conditions where particular genetic predispositions make the selection of certain medications more likely to have better outcomes.

Two similar patients, for all their similarities, still may not have the same response to the same drug, depending on differences in their genetic makeup. The more we understand individual genetic codes and the more variables we can gather and analyze, the better we will be able to select the right treatment and exactly the right drug. In the future, as we understand the genetic makeup of each individual and learn more about genes on an individual level, we will be able to target medications and treatments based on each individual's makeup and response.

Using AI in Treatment

By now, you know to anticipate my claim about the tremendous benefits that AI might provide in this area. My primary claim is this: AI can be used to determine, based on the specifics of a given case, which treatment has the highest likelihood of being most effective or delivering the most positive outcome for a particular patient. That means AI could help physicians determine which medication or approach is the very best one for treating an individual patient—namely, which medication will most likely help *this* person, given *this* combination of conditions, under *these* specific circumstances, at *this* given moment.

Here are some ways that might play out.

SELECTING MORE SUCCESSFUL TREATMENTS

One way we might use machine learning in treatment selection is to allow machines to teach themselves about what has been the case so far. Machines could look at a large number of patients, all the treatments they experienced, all the medication that they took, and then look at their outcomes, both at key points during treatment and at their final outcomes. Far more easily than a human brain, AI can review patient characteristics, various drugs, dosages, regimens and protocols, and the ultimate outcome for those processes. A machine learning algorithm *can see the route for the patient*, the path, the drug, the protocol, and the dosage. Right now, the way medicine is practiced, we are not able to fine-tune a treatment for a patient in that way.

At the very least, and sooner rather than later, we could intervene in the process of prioritizing treatments if we could simply predict which drug is likely to have the most positive effect on the patient. Instead of a trial and error process that is time consuming, expensive, and potentially harmful to a patient, whatever drug is predicted to be a best match could be the first drug tried. We could target the right drug for the patient *on the first attempt.*

In cases requiring complicated protocols for all the interventions that have to occur, AI would allow the data to guide the protocol. Let me explain. Let's say there are six interventions that need to be done to treat a particular disease, and all six are necessary. Let's also say that each of those interventions is either a medicine or a procedure. We know already how this has played out using the traditional model. A particular scientist who is a specialist in one area will test a protocol on a group of patients and advise that in order to treat this condition, the physician and patients will need to do A, B, C, D, E, F in the following order and combination. We know already that running these studies and sharing their results can take quite some time, and we know that protocols tested on small groups do not always have the same effects when they are used in a broad population.

These are just the kinds of study that can be done not only differently but more quickly, efficiently, and precisely, using AI. Machine learning can quickly figure out which components of a protocol actually work and which components do not contribute to positive outcomes. And because not every component may be valuable in all patients, when we add information specific to each patient, only those components of the protocol that will make a difference in a specific patient are the ones that would be utilized.

TRACKING PATIENT RESPONSE
TO TREATMENT

As discussed in the example of sepsis in the previous chapter, AI can carry out an analysis of patient response to treatment *in real time.* For example, the National Institutes of Health (NIH) created an app to monitor patients' medication regimens.[21] Through the app, AI can confirm that patients are or are not taking their prescription medicines. This helps patients stay on track and can help doctors quickly spot those patients who may need additional assistance adhering to a treatment protocol.

Assisting with Surgery and Recovery

Finally, AI can actually intervene in treatment processes, including assisting doctors with surgery and tracking patients' recovery after they return home from the hospital setting. Again, work sponsored by the NIH shows that AI algorithms can enhance surgical precision—for example, by "seeing" tumor margin cells that are invisible to surgeons or by finding the least disruptive pathway for reaching tumors in high-risk locations that are difficult to reach.[22]

Those are the types of advantages that a machine learning algorithm can offer and that can take us all the way from prediction to diagnosis to treatment with greater accuracy, greater savings, and better health outcomes. Imagine going from being able to better predict who will get breast cancer to better determining how frequently their mammograms need to be done, to being able to determine whether a particular patient should pursue surgery, chemotherapy, or other treatments. Given what we know about the

---

21 Novatio Solutions, "Ten Common Applications of Artificial Intelligence in Healthcare," *Novatio* blog post, 2018, https://novatiosolutions.com/10-common-applications-artificial-intelligence-healthcare.

22 Blake Hannaford, "The Marriage of Artificial Intelligence and Patient Care," Media Planet, Future of Business and Tech editorial, http://www.futureofbusinessandtech.com/business-solutions/the-marriage-of-artificial-intelligence-and-patient-care.

treatment benefits of an early diagnosis, we can already imagine patients benefiting from less aggressive or less physically destructive and less painful treatments as a result of AI's knowledge, accuracy, and speed in identifying tumors, including ones that the human eye might not catch. Aggressive treatment would not have to be contemplated except for those patients whose disease situation truly warrants such treatment. If there is one thing that's currently true of the public imagination about cancers right now, it's the assumption that if the cancer itself doesn't kill the patient, the treatment eventually will. The cancer treatment process, in particular, would be well served by the identification of drugs and protocols that did not have to be as destructive are they are currently.

SOLVING TREATMENT DILEMMAS

I want to look quickly at one other example in this chapter, before we dig deeper into the application of AI in treatment scenarios in the next. I'm going out on a limb with this example, as it is a hot political issue and one that seems impossible for the health care community to address either directly or sufficiently.

The problem I want to consider is opiate addiction. Essentially, opiates have become a predominant part of treatment plans for surgery, injury, or for other bodily traumas. Of 100 surgery patients who have never before taken opiates, which their doctor is now prescribing for them—hydrocodone, for example—13 percent will become hooked on the opiates if they take them for more than five days, as recommended by their doctor. Thirteen percent of them will become hooked *in just five days*.[23] Even patients who haven't had

---

23   A. Shah, C. J. Hayes, and B. C. Martin, "Characteristics of Initial Prescription
      Episodes and Likelihood of Long-Term Opioid Use: United States, 2006–2015,"
      Morbidity and Mortality Weekly Report (*MMWR*) 66, no. 10 (March 17, 2017):
      265–269, https://dx.doi.org/10.15585/mmwr.mm6610a1.

surgery but who simply stay in the hospital for a few days and are given narcotic pain medicine, can also get hooked. Opiates can be that dangerous.

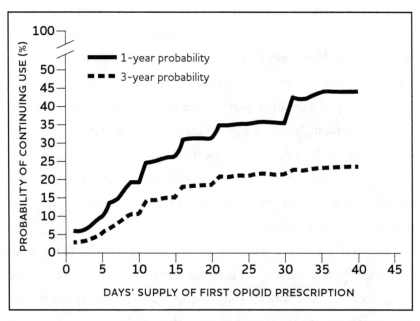

One- and three-year probabilities of continued opioid use among opioid-naïve patients by number of days' supply of the first opioid prescription—United States, 2006–2015. Source: Anuj Shah, Corey J. Hayes, and Bradley C. Martin, *Morbidity and Mortality Weekly Report*, Centers for Disease Control and Prevention, March 17, 2017, https://www.cdc.gov/mmwr/volumes/66/wr/mm6610a1.htm.

Opioid usage has become such a major menace in the United States that while this country makes up only 5 percent of the world population, its citizens consume nearly 80 percent of the world's opioid drugs.[24] We end up with a vicious cycle in which people become hooked on narcotics and become long-term users, turning to higher and higher dosages in order to address their pain. Eventually, they turn to dangerous illegal drugs—shooting heroin, for example— to keep up with their addiction. That's how people die. According

24   Dina Gusovsky, "Americans Still Lead the World in Something: Use of Highly Addictive Opioids," CNBC, April 27, 2016.

to the Centers for Disease Control (CDC), in 2016 alone, around forty-six people died *every day* from overdoses involving prescription opioids.[25]

Not only are narcotics dangerously addictive but their addictive quality contributes to lowering a person's pain threshold so that patients *actually hurt more when they are taking the medicine than they would if they were not on the narcotic*. Patients taking narcotics can start to feel pains in other parts of the body and will crave more of the narcotic medicine. In a way, taking narcotic pain medicines does a disservice to the body; as the pain threshold keeps decreasing, it becomes harder to control. Between physical dependence and psychological dependence, the threat presented by narcotics would seem to outweigh the benefits.

On the one hand, we have achieved longevity in the human lifespan. People are living longer, and everything would seem to be going well. On the other hand, one of the big reasons people are dying prematurely is drug addiction. Part of the reason for this is that we've come to think of narcotics as the sole solution for pain. But there are other medications that work just as well as narcotics, sometimes even better, and they don't cause a feeling of euphoria, that can be addictive. The hard truth may be that narcotics *are not essential.* What if physicians prescribed narcotics only for patients who are dying of cancer or during end of life?

The first question we should ask ourselves is how we failed to know this effect of narcotics, when narcotics have been used in clinical treatment for more than a century. The answer is that we never looked. We should ask why some people get hooked and others don't. Why do 13 percent of patients on opioids get hooked and become long-term

---

25   Centers for Disease Control and Prevention, "Prescription Opioid Data," *Opioid Overdose,* last updated August 30, 2017, https://www.cdc.gov/drugoverdose/data/overdose.html.

users? And now we can also ask whether there is a way to tell if patients can become narcotic dependent *before* we prescribe them narcotics. Are there certain tendencies? Are there certain markers? Are there certain characteristics, or previous life experiences, or even previous drug experiences that contribute to their chances?

As we consider the value of narcotics for treating pain in patients who are not dying, AI allows us realistically to ask whether we could predict, by way of physical and psychological assessments, who will have a negative outcome from using opioids. Could we avoid using narcotics in the first place for those people who are at high risk for becoming addicted? Machine learning offers us the opportunity to determine which factors go into the formula to determine who makes an ideal candidate for narcotic abuse. If we can identify those early on, maybe we can prevent the disaster of addiction from happening to individuals later in life. Maybe that would also help us alert more people, innocent people who don't know that opioid addiction can so easily happen to them. And if the possibility of making this determination exists, shouldn't we be working right now toward rescuing people from the threat of addiction and an early death?

Overall Benefits

I'll end here, as I have in previous chapters, with a brief review of the treatment benefits of AI to the three groups we've been considering along the way: doctors, companies, and patients.

Doctors can utilize AI to determine best treatment plans and medications, because AI can bring to bear tremendous amounts of data— from disease-specific data to patient-specific data—for the treatment of a single patient. AI can put the accumulated knowledge of doctors all over the world at the service of any given doctor in any given location, and it can assess new and emerging treatments better and faster than clinical trials can. The pattern-recognition abilities of AI can catch details and find connections that no human or team of humans could find as quickly. This can help doctors predict disease, spot the earliest signs of disease, and begin appropriate treatments sooner.

Companies that fund health care for their employees are under tremendous financial pressure due to the rising cost of health care and the damage illness causes to their workers. Health care companies that are really trying to do the right thing, identifying disease early and accurately and treating conditions efficiently, will see the benefit of AI in assisting their mission. Use of AI can save billions of dollars wasted each year on treatments that may be unnecessary, as well as those that turn out to be unhelpful or even dangerous.

Patients will experience decreased illness burden. They will save time and money, but most importantly, they stand to benefit from the prevention of exposure to harmful side effects and from early initiation to truly helpful treatment plans. AI can help customize treatment plans for individuals by recognizing all the ways that the same drug can have vastly different effects and outcomes in different people. AI can offer patients the best chance of surviving longer and maintaining the best possible quality of life when facing cancers and other life-threatening illnesses. And AI could make it so that people have access to the therapies they need in the places where they live, without having to travel from their hometowns to areas of the country or the world where a particular treatment is available.

CHAPTER 7

Treatment:
The Application

n this chapter, I want to consider a few examples of ways that AI can assist clinicians in the treatment process—from contributing details about patients and conditions to the determination of whether, when, and which kinds of intervention are needed, to providing up-to-the-minute information that can simplify participation in clinical trials of new medications and procedures. The utilization of AI can help determine the best steps forward for particular patients at many points in the disease treatment processes. In doing so, AI can dramatically increase the effectiveness and maintenance of that process.

Surgeries

Surgeries have been considered to be the definitive treatment for a number of health problems. For example, tonsillectomies were once a common procedure to treat tonsil inflammation and infection. Patients who had an infection in their tonsils went to their doctor who gave them antibiotics and scheduled them for surgery. The idea of surgery as a necessary component of treatment is still the norm with procedures such as hysterectomies to treat fibroids and endometriosis, caesarian sections to address a sluggish labor, and cholecystectomy to relieve gall bladder symptoms.

These surgeries are not minor ones. Besides the fact that surgeries are costly, there are also always potential complications and consequences that should not be taken lightly. Furthermore, we are learning that surgery may not be necessary in many cases. In the case of tonsils, for instance, it may not even be helpful for patients to have them removed. It turns out patients may need their tonsils in order to be capable in the long term of fighting infections and sustaining immunity to certain illnesses.

Surgeries such as the ones I mention here raise some questions. How should we select patients who will benefit from a particular surgery, and how do we know which ones will not really benefit? At the very least, we should be able to make three clear categorizations in evaluating the need for surgery: people who will benefit from surgery, people who will benefit from antibiotics or other medicines and treatment plans without surgery, and people for whom neither medicines nor surgery are necessary.

Let's take the example of a child who comes into a hospital's emergency services with severe belly pain that turns out to be appendicitis. Normally, the treatment would automatically be surgery and at least one overnight stay in the hospital. However, a significant portion of appendicitis patients can be successfully treated with antibiotics, making the surgery and hospital stay unnecessary. What if there were a tool that could predict which patients are most likely to have positive outcomes on antibiotics alone, without undergoing surgery and its complications? I want to suggest that with enough data, an AI system could reliably provide this information.

In part, predicting who might be able to avoid surgery for appendicitis hinges on being able to tell whether or not an appendix is likely to burst. We absolutely want to avoid the appendix bursting and making a mess in the abdomen. Abdominal infection can lead to complications in the short term and long-term damage in the abdomen. Because the appendix is connected to the colon, the abdomen usually becomes contaminated with stool. Additionally, as with any surgery, the potential exists for complications from anesthesia, from infection, and from bleeding to occur. Then there are the costs of surgery, hospitalization, use of the operating room, and care in the clinic, as well as complications, such as hospital-acquired infections that are difficult to treat. All those things add up for the patient. Because antibiotics do help in resolving appendicitis, at least in selected cases, if there is a way to predict and select the candidates who would recover with antibiotics versus those who need surgery, we could prevent patients having to go under the knife.

Trying to identify those candidates would mean determining relevant characteristics of both patient and appendix. Do patients have to be a certain age? Does the appendix have to be a certain size, a certain shape, a certain length, or a certain width? Do we look for certain consistencies on the CT scan? These are all questions that we haven't yet studied and that physicians may be able to use AI to answer. To be able to answer some of these questions would help us know which patients definitely need surgery and which ones might safely be treated conservatively, with antibiotics and other alternatives.

Right now, though, every time someone comes in with a case of appendicitis, the protocol is to err on the side of caution and do the surgery. And even now, with all the technology that is available—the ultrasounds, the CT scans, the blood tests—there is still a certain rate of rupture. That rate of rupture is about 30 percent. It has decreased, but not much, over time, even as the scans and other technologies have improved.[26] Before there were CTs, physicians would just feel the belly and do a blood test, and then determine whether or not the patient had appendicitis. Now, CTs allow us to see the appendix better than ever before, and yet that rate of rupture still remains pretty high.

Some might argue that it is better to err on the side of caution and remove the infected appendix. There are two problems with erring on the side of caution, however, and these two problems lie on opposite ends of the spectrum. One complication, as we know already, is the event of rupture, when the appendix bursts before it can be treated or removed. This is the case of the false negative, when the conditions indicating rupture are missed. The other complication is the false positive: patients have all the symptoms and signs, including tests that all indicate appendicitis. So, physicians take them to the operating room, open them up, take out the appendix, and send it to the pathology lab, which reports that there is no inflammation, no infection, anywhere in the appendix. In the first case, the treatment should have happened early enough to avoid the event of bursting. In the second case, the treatment did not need to occur.

By setting a machine the task of studying just these two opposite types of problem, we might be able to figure out the characteristics of those patients whose appendices burst and the characteristics of those patients who have a perfectly normal appendix, despite seeming to be

---

26   M. L. Barrett, A. L. Hines, and R. M. Andrews, "Trends in Rates of Perforated Appendix, 2001–2010," Statistical Brief #159, Agency for Health care Quality Research, Health Care Cost and Utilization Project, July 2013, https://www. hcup-us.ahrq.gov/reports/statbriefs/sb159.pdf; A. B. Kharbanda et al., "Development and Validation of a Novel Pediatric Appendicitis Calculator (pARC)," Pediatrics 141, no. 4 (April 2018), https://doi.org/10.1542/peds.2017-2699.

infected. Given the capabilities that AI has already proven to have, it's easy to imagine that a machine might give us an answer, potentially saving patients with appendicitis from further complications in their condition and saving patients without appendicitis from unnecessary surgeries. In between these two ends of the spectrum, AI might also help us determine which patients are better candidates for surgery and which may benefit fully from a course of antibiotics and a wait-and-see approach.

Decision Support

We began this chapter by looking forward to a future use of AI in determining treatment, preventing unnecessary surgeries, and better guarding against situations that would make surgery risky and outcomes worse. But now let's consider an example of AI as it is currently being put to use in the ICU.

Remember that, in the ICU, a variety of data is being continuously collected. This trove of information can be used to track subtle trends in patient status and make predictions about their stability. Remember, too, that CDSSs are the tools used to make these predictions and evaluate the severity of a patient's condition.

The idea here is that a CDSS will help predict which patients are going to get worse and will need a higher level of care. The CDSSs currently in use deliver less-than-ideal results. In fact, they can fail to identify nearly 60 percent of unstable patients in some cases. As a result, each year, patient transfer and discharge errors cost billions of dollars and lead to at least forty-six thousand deaths that might have been prevented.

One limitation of the existing CDSS tools is that they may treat risk factors independently of one another. These tools are not particularly sensitive to the relationships among or between risk factors. This means that patients often don't get needed care in the right care setting until it's too late. If hospitals had better tools for tracking the relationships among risk factors, they could improve treatment significantly.

Let me tell you about an AI tool that does just that. It is called AutoTriage, and because of its sensitivity to subtle imbalances in patient status, it helps predict patient instability and mortality and can even help forecast other patient outcomes that are less dire. Being able to predict these changes in the ICU is absolutely critical for making timely interventions, for managing patient needs, and for using limited resources to maximum benefit. Essentially, AutoTriage improves physicians' ability to predict in-hospital death, making it possible to intervene early on in more efficient and effective ways than before.

Let me give you a little more detail about how the system improves the CDSSs that predict patient stability and mortality in the ICU. By now you will not be surprised that part of the success of AutoTriage comes from its reliance on the widely available EHR data. When utilized to their full capacity, EHRs really do provide an opportunity to use medical information for more accurate patient care. The algorithm for AutoTriage uses eight very common clinical variables from the EHR to assign patient mortality risk scores. Each variable has its own score, as do specific combinations of variables. The overall score combines all the variables.[27]

It is true that the current CDSSs do already account for variables such as patient age, type of admission, and vital signs. But what AutoTriage does, quite simply, is carefully analyze the relationships among

27   J. Calvert et al., "Using Electronic Health Record Collected Clinical Variables to Predict Medical Intensive Care Unit Mortality," *Annals of Medicine and Surgery* 11 (November 2016): 52–57, https://doi.org/10.1016/j.amsu.2016.09.002.

the variables. I say "simply" because it seems so obvious that considering the relationships among and between risk factors would make for greater sensitivity to the actual and complex physiology of patients. But the current systems just aren't capable of making those connections. They're also not capable of accounting for individual patient differences, or for real-time trends in patient vital signs. By looking at information about patient status, and by analyzing correlations and trends, AutoTriage provides far more accurate information about patient stability.

Comparison of *AutoTriage* performance with commonly used disease severity scores for the prediction of 12 h mortality in the Medical Intensive Care Unit. *PPV* = positive predictive value, *NPV* = negative predictive value, *DOR* = diagnostic odds ratio. *SAPS II* = Simplified Acute Physiology Score, *SOFA* = Sequential Organ Failure Assessment, *MEWS* = Modified Early Warning Score.

	AutoTriage ($\geq$ -2)	*SAPS II* ($\geq$ 21)	*SOFA* ($\geq$ 6)	*MEWS* ($\geq$ 2)	*MEWS* ($\geq$ 3)
AUROC	0.88	0.71	0.72	0.75	0.75
Sensitivity	0.80	0.76	0.76	0.78	0.66
Specificity	0.81	0.51	0.53	0.59	0.74
PPV	0.44	0.23	0.24	0.27	0.33
NPV	0.95	0.92	0.92	0.93	0.92
DOR	16.26	3.35	3.59	5.01	5.41
Accuracy	0.80	0.55	0.57	0.62	0.73

Source: Jacob Calvert, "Using electronic health record collected clinical variables to predict medical intensive care unit mortality," Annals of Medicine and Surgery 11 (2016): 52–57, https://doi.org/10.1016/j.amsu.2016.09.002.

Progress Treating Cancers

In the previous chapter, we talked about how complex and difficult it is to generate a treatment protocol for each individual patient. Of course, there are guidelines, and these are updated often because the science changes so fast. Even with the guidelines, to be able to digest all the clinical data and then come up with a solution has become extremely challenging.

For any doctor, the exponential growth of clinical information makes for an uphill battle to get a handle on the data needed to optimize patient outcomes. For an oncologist practicing in an under-resourced hospital to be able to stay abreast of the science and determine a comprehensive plan for each patient, it is even more difficult. Oftentimes, patients will be sent to bigger hospitals, mainly because the larger hospitals tend to have more cancer experience overall. But for the community hospital oncologist especially, it can take a long time, easily several days, before a treatment plan can be initiated.

Typically, what happens is that the physician sees a patient and determines what stage the cancer is at and whether it has spread to other organs or not. Then the physician devises a treatment plan. Most cases then go before what is called a tumor board comprised of specialists: oncologists, surgeons, radiation therapists, chemo doctors, and pharmacists. All these people, ten to fifteen or so, sit together and review individual cases and help come up with or verify a treatment plan. The treatment plan can be anywhere from surgery, to chemotherapy, radiation therapy, and/or palliative treatment. Palliative treatment occurs when no existing plan of attack is thought to be useful to the patient. Depending on the patient's wishes, palliative care focuses on treating and managing symptoms and not necessarily on curing the cancer. But even in palliative cases, there are still palliative-oriented surgeries, radiation, and so forth.

My overall point is this: a lot of effort and a lot of time go into the determination of the treatment.

Making sure that patients get the best possible care available to them, improving care overall, and making sure that information about treatment is distributed widely is already being addressed by a team at Memorial Sloan Kettering Cancer Center (MSK) in New York, in collaboration with IBM Watson. So far, they've developed two key products for providing treatment recommendations.

One of these products matches patients to clinical trials. It operates by analyzing patient genomes and addresses the issue of physicians not being able to track the sheer number, let alone all the details, of rapidly emerging therapies. This product analyzes large amounts of data in a systematic way and helps doctors make that information meaningful in an individual patient case. The additional benefit to cancer science and patient health is that the more patients are enrolled in clinical trials, the faster our understanding and actual treatment procedures will materialize. Instead of researchers having to wait for a certain number of patients to enroll in their studies, researchers can get patients faster, finish trials sooner, and have answers that can then be refined and implemented in further treatment of the disease.

Even though there is an insurance requirement for people to have access to clinical trials, right now, only 5 percent of the patients being treated for cancer actually do enroll in those trials. In other words, *the demand for access to trials far exceeds the actual record of access.* Most patients don't enroll because they are unaware of trials that are available to them, and sometimes they are equally unaware of the full range of drugs and treatment that are available for a specific type of cancer.

The number of treatment options for patients is growing rapidly, especially in terms of identifying genetic markers—which show us the possibility of a patient developing a particular cancer and which suggests the appropriate means of treating that cancer—and growing the field of immuno-oncology. Linking more patients to appropriate trials has the potential to help patients currently suffering from cancer and advance the science that will help even more patients in the future.

The second product the MSK-IBM team has developed is a machine that processes information from myriad sources—medical literature, medical records, imaging, lab, and pathology reports, existing treatment guidelines, and the collective knowledge of experts at MSK—in order to help make recommendations for individual therapies.[28] In other words, the machine creates a treatment protocol from the accumulated knowledge to which it is given access. To test this function, researchers compared the machine's treatment recommendations to those of the tumor board. The treatments recommended by both the board and the Watson machine were very similar, the two agreeing 80 percent or more of the time. That means that this new technology can help doctors make better evidence-based treatment decisions with far greater speed than has been the case to date.

Essentially, the machine serves as a clinical decision board system. It offers three recommendations: a green light, a yellow, and a red. The green light conveys the message that any of these drugs can be given and it recommends the drug of choice. Yellow conveys the recommendation that a certain drug could be tried. Red warns that a certain drug or treatment should not be used. The *speed* with which Watson operates is something that we've come to expect from

---

28 S. P. Somashekhar et al. "Early Experience with IBM Watson for Oncology (WFO) Cognitive Computing System for Lung and Colorectal Cancer Treatment," *Journal of Clinical Oncology* 35, no. 15 (May 20, 2017 supplement): 8527, doi: 10.1200/ JCO.2017.35.15_suppl.8527.

a machine, but the *accuracy* of the machine's findings and treatment recommendations is a clear reflection of the extreme benefit of this sort of technology. Let's not forget, either, that this particular technology was developed in a large cancer center where the information fed to it reflects a tremendous amount of accumulated experience and knowledge. To be able take those large amounts of accumulated experience and knowledge and analyze them in detail is the real contribution of AI in this setting.

I want to emphasize that *one needs a very high level of expertise to be able to recommend a cancer treatment.* So, when a machine shows the capacity to match a tumor board, we are not just talking about machines being able to do an okay job. We're talking about them quickly developing a level of expertise that is capable, minimally, of matching the knowledge accumulated by many human experts.

Let's not forget, too, that our current sets of general guidelines are just that: generalized recommendations assembled by entities such as the American Society of Clinical Oncology and similar organizations. These guidelines can only go so far, which means that they tend to remain more generic than they could be. For them to better reflect the differences in each patient, we need to utilize an analytical system with the abilities that only AI can provide.

I think it's important to mention two limitations of the projects that I've addressed here. One is that in the second study, the machine did not develop novel protocols. Right now, the machine's capacity is to analyze and select from what is fed to it rather than to generate new knowledge. In other words, the researchers have not yet leveraged the biggest asset in machine learning and AI—namely, tracking the outcomes of machine recommendations in order to use that information for a more granular and more individual-specific approach to cancer treatment.

The second limitation is a transparency issue. When a machine comes up with a recommendation, the treating physician may not be able to tell why the machine picked that treatment. This is called a black box problem. The machine does all its calculations, but the physician may have no way of telling why the machine is recommending Treatment A over Treatment B. One of the things that researchers are working on now is coming up with a way to make that process transparent so that the physician can actually see why the machine picked a certain treatment or why it is recommending a certain pathway.

Though these are limitations, they are merely temporary ones. Their solutions are clearly within reach and should be thought of as indications of how well and quickly we will be able to develop the capacity of AI systems to help us solve increasingly complicated health problems.

CANCER AS A FOCUS AREA FOR AI

Increasing longevity within the world's population is contributing to the higher prevalence of cancer worldwide. Heart disease and stroke still are, in most places, the number-one killers. But the very application of the preventive measures that we discussed early on in this book—managing diabetes, high blood pressure, cholesterol, smoking, and so on—have the effect of decreasing the death rate from cardiovascular disease. What is happening is that cancer is taking over, especially among the older population, as a number-one killer. It is reasonable to predict that as time goes on and prevention for heart disease and a number of other diseases continues to succeed, people will live longer, and there will be more cancers. We will increasingly need machines with the ability to help predict, diagnose, and treat cancers in order to address their increased occurrence.

DRUG DEVELOPMENT

One final word about how AI technology might assist with cancer treatment is that it can help pick the candidates for drug development—the molecules and the types of combinations of molecules or even drugs that have been used for other diseases and that might work in a particular case—*without actually having to conduct a clinical experiment to do so.* This is a fascinating area of current research. With the help of AI technologies, scientists can go through thousands of molecules of new potential drugs and run experiments online without necessarily using those molecules on patients.[29] This process helps them narrow the options to a smaller set of promising molecules, so that they might test only the ones with the highest likelihood of success against a certain disease.

Lung cancer is the most common type of cancer in the world, killing more than a million people annually. There are two types of lung cancers: non-small-cell lung cancer, which is the most common type (80 percent) and the more dreaded small cell lung cancer. The small cell lung cancer spreads rapidly and kills its victims in a matter of weeks to months with no known cure. With the availability of large amounts of data and machine learning technologies, it is possible to search for treatments that may be useful in treating this type of lung cancer. In fact, a group of researchers who are involved in this type of research found out that a commonly used antidepressant medication may be useful in treating small cell lung cancer! This was done just by researching the data to find correlations. Later scientists were able

---

29   Nadine S. Jahchan, "A Drug Repositioning Approach Identifies Tricyclic Antidepressants as Inhibitors of Small Cell Lung Cancer and Other Neuroendocrine Tumors," *Cancer Discovery* 3, no. 12 (December 10, 2013): 1364–1377, https://www.ncbi.nlm.nih.gov/pmc/articles/PMC3864571; Adriana Zingone et al., "Relationship between Anti-Depressant Use and Lung Cancer Survival," *Cancer Treatment and Research Communications* 10 (2017): 33–39, https://www.ncbi.nlm.nih.gov/pmc/articles/PMC5603309.

to find out that this was in fact true in real patients.

The potential for using AI in cancer drug development is tremendous. As we well know, one of the problems with drug development is that it takes a very long time, time that most cancer patients do not have. It can also be an expensive endeavor. A new drug can take, on average, ten years and $2 billion to get from discovery to market. Compressing that period using new AI technologies could really open up the options for more successful forms of cancer treatment and extend patients' lives.

CHAPTER 8

Fulfilling a Promise

I n a village in an ancient, peaceful Indian kingdom, there was a great temple. People from near and far sought out this temple for worship and to celebrate momentous occasions in their lives.

Eventually, forces came and defeated the king who had ruled over the village and the temple. The king lost his kingdom and his life, and the village and its temple were looted. Its inhabitants were left destitute and without protection.

But there remained a secret that only the surviving villagers knew. Generations of kings had stored their treasures and wealth—gold, jewels, monies from around the globe—in a vault hidden under the temple. Knowledge of this secret presented the villagers with the opportunity to conquer their poverty and renew their lives.

However, the legend surrounding the temple warned that whoever opened the doors to the treasure would be cursed with long suffering. For this reason, knowing of the treasure and of the legend surrounding it, the villagers continued to live in poverty, without food to eat and without the means to care sufficiently for their young and their elderly. They stayed in the village, all the while knowing that buried beneath the temple was a treasure that could save and vastly improve their lives. They suffered famine and many of them perished. Those who lived, knowing both of the treasure and the curse, did not dare enter the temple vault for fear that it might cause them greater woe than they already suffered.

This story, in all its drama, relates quite well to the current state of health care in the United States.

Let me explain. I've talked a lot in this book about the EHR. I have pointed out that we have a wealth of data in the EHR that we are not yet really able to access, let alone put to good use. This data could throw light on so much that we don't yet understand. It could significantly improve our ability to diagnose and treat patients and it could enable us to deliver truly patient-centric care. This information could offer clues on how to prevent disease. The basis of our ability to save ourselves is hidden, like a buried treasure, in the EHRs and other clinical data repositories.

Just as in the story of the ancient village, there is a curse keeping us from accessing these stores of accumulated wealth. What's the fearful curse keeping us from taking advantage of the data that we have stored away?

There are many forces influencing health care delivery that are driven by the fear of losing money. This fear is something I've hinted at by pointing out the abundance of waste in health care. Were we to acknowledge that there are procedures, tests, medicines, and treatment plans that are useless, the elimination of those useless things would mean the loss of money for health care organizations and job loss or job changes for certain health care professionals. Concerns over changed job responsibilities, over eliminated work, and over profits and losses have perverted current assumptions about the use of AI in health care practice. These concerns keep us from moving forward in the direction of improving our lot overall.

Health care has overtaken retail as the biggest employer in the United States.[30] And when politicians talk about expanding health care even more, they are signaling the creation of even more jobs. They promise more jobs, knowing that the addition of those jobs forces us to sustain a system based on inefficiency and ridiculous spending.

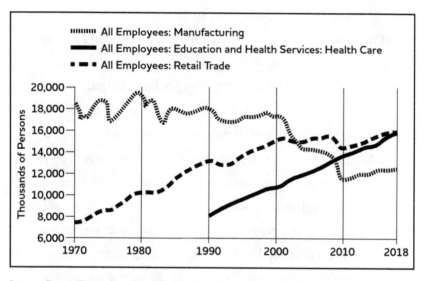

Source: Derek Thompson, "Health Care Just Became the U.S.'s Largest Employer," *The Atlantic*, January 9, 2018, https://www.theatlantic.com/business/archive/2018/01/health-care-america-jobs/550079.

Many suppliers and employers also fear outcomes-based research because of the real possibility that their businesses will be hurt by its findings. Hospitals worry that they will not be able to profit by filling hospital beds. Radiologists and pathologists worry their jobs will be taken over by machines. Surgeons worry that fewer of them will be necessary should the procedures in which they specialize be needed less often. Companies that provide drugs, devices, and other

30   Derek Thompson, "Health Care Just Became the U.S.'s Largest Employer," *The Atlantic*, January 9, 2018, https://www.theatlantic.com/business/archive/2018/01/health-care-america-jobs/550079/.

equipment worry about their products becoming obsolete.

In light of all these fears, how might we make the case for moving all our lives forward, for accessing the buried treasure and accepting the consequences of the "curse" of job and profit losses that we imagine will destroy us, or at least destroy our health care system? Can we even make a convincing argument that the benefits for our primary stakeholders—patients, doctors, and companies—are all worth the risk, or worth the projected costs of changing course?

Let me suggest, first, that the burden set upon us by our current system of health care is not being fully acknowledged. We are not altogether aware of the extent to which we, in the United States, are like the villagers who were suffering from famine and yet unwilling to risk saving their own lives. Raising awareness of our real situation, of its dangerous inefficiency, is one part of addressing our fears.

We might begin with companies that spend inordinate amounts of money to provide health insurance for their employees. General Motors has been described as being in the health care business rather than the automotive business because the company spends more on providing health care than it does on purchasing steel to manufacture its cars. Starbucks, too, spends more money on health care than on purchasing coffee beans![31]

Can we convince employers that there are ways of spending less on health care, while having a healthier workforce, higher employee productivity, and sustaining or even growing company outputs?

Similarly, we might pay more attention to patient expenses. Can we convince patients that it would be best to have a system that wouldn't bankrupt them when they faced serious health conditions or needed hospitalization or medication?

---

31 Dave Chase, "You Run a Health-Care Business Whether You Like It or Not," CFO, November 7. 2017, http://ww2.cfo.com/health-benefits/2017/11/run-health-care-business-whether-like-not.

That these questions seem easily answered by a yes brings to the fore how ludicrous it is for a company or for a patient to reject clear benefits to each of them: lowered costs, better and more precise care, and the potential for overall health to improve.

And so, it must be that the fear of the "curse" of losing out belongs primarily to the business of health care itself, to those who control health care agencies: the pharmaceutical companies, the medical device companies, the hospitals, and those who are employed as health care professionals. Worrying over changed job responsibility and job loss in certain sectors of the health care industry is essentially, and perversely, to value employment more than health. It is to prefer unhealthy people and more jobs to healthy people and potentially fewer jobs. The same is, of course, true for the industry as a whole: profit is valued more than increased or sustained well-being.

In chapter 4, I mentioned the issue of doctors hesitating to embrace new technologies, but that is only true of *some* doctors, not all. After all, doctors, as a whole, have always been on the front end of experimenting with and utilizing new technologies and implementing new ways of doing things. That is part of what it means to participate in a field with an ever-expanding knowledge base. Might some doctors' jobs change as a result of the widespread use of AI in clinical practice? Yes. Will there be a decrease in certain kinds of work that doctors currently do? Yes. Likely, as we discussed in that earlier chapter, this change would be a reduction in the most mundane and repetitive tasks. Reducing those tasks (automating triage processes, for example) could lead doctors to re-envision their profession, to see what more and what else can be done. But doctors will be able to function on a much higher level.

The aid provided by machines in alleviating certain responsibilities invites doctors to entertain yet other responsibilities. As with any new technologies, machine learning and artificial intelligence present us with the opportunity to utilize them as we see fit. They give us a way of making work more efficient, of making outcomes better, and of devoting our time and energy to the parts of the process that matter most.

I would emphasize that there are so many aspects of scientific understanding, of human intelligence, and of human skill that simply cannot be replaced by machines. In fact, all of the examples we have discussed in this book have been about the use of AI as an *assistive* technology. That implies that there's always a need for human supervision and control of machines. Patients, too, will always need there to be a human presence. Someone who can understand, decipher, correct, and adjust treatment plans and customize them to specific patients, and someone who does all of these tasks *with knowledge from lived experience that machines don't have the capacity to decipher.*

I cannot emphasize this enough: beyond technicalities, and in a way that incorporates those technicalities, there will always be a need for doctors to think carefully about patient care and to demonstrate compassion, understanding, empathy, trustworthiness—all those human behaviors that patients need and rely on for both their mental and physical well-being. Plenty of aspects of care will still have to be carried out by real human physicians, and this will continue to have the highest value for patients, both physically and psychologically. The ability of machines to analyze numeric variables or pixel patterns doesn't even touch on the capacities for human modulation that are so necessary to good health care.

Machines also are not able to carry out the very human work of determining causation. The role of researchers is likely to change, given that machine learning can study outcomes in an entire population. But what machine learning shows us is *correlations*. To be able to confirm those correlations and figure out what is causing them will still be necessary human work. Performing clinical trials to test this technology will still be a human function. The same is true for determining which tasks will be carried out by machines, how they will be carried out, and how they will be monitored and improved. There will be a much bigger role for physician-scientists in monitoring AI systems and processes, in making sure that the machines are working as intended, and in fine-tuning algorithms for the sake of more careful or more targeted study. There will be a new subspecialty in medicine dealing with data science.

The assistive nature of AI will set up doctors to have more meaningful interactions with patients, and it will also help doctors reach patients for whom they could not otherwise provide care. Tracking patients with AI technologies can decrease the need for clinic visits and allow doctors to take care of some patients remotely. More people might receive appropriate care if they did not have to arrange transportation to the doctor's office each time they needed assistance. Doctors could have more direct contact with their patients, as monitoring a patient via an AI system decreases the need for intermediaries transferring information back and forth between physician and patient. Interaction with a physician could be enhanced rather than reduced by expansions of the "space" of the clinic that AI could make possible.

Moving Forward

Right now, most doctors don't have on hand the sorts of AI tools we've been discussing in this book. There are at least three components that would have to belong to any sustainable plan for putting AI technology in the hands of practicing physicians.

- First, we need continuous development of the technology itself; truly, we have just scratched the surface of what is possible.

- Second, clinician-scientists need training in AI technologies and access to the wealth of clinical data.

- Third, we need to grow the number of talented people who have the cross-disciplinary knowledge to develop and make use of both the technology and the data.

Some of these goals should be relatively easy to achieve. For example, for the *technology* that is already out there, organizations simply need the ability to procure it. And since most organizations already use EHRs, the *data* is, at least in one sense, also already there. As I see it, the biggest challenge is finding and cultivating the *talent*, the people specifically trained to manage, manipulate, and devise solutions from all the information that's available. Ideally, the right people for the job are those who understand both data science and health care: physician-researchers who can move so easily within these two areas that they can see the means of merging the two successfully. As we move forward and as available data and knowledge continue to increase, we will have to rely more and more on teams that can design applications and deliver information to physicians in real time and at the point of care—when they're seeing patients during appointments—and in ways that are immediately useful to both doctors and patients in that setting.

The transformation within health care to becoming a more data-driven, digital enterprise has been happening very slowly. It is a transformation that is happening with greater speed in other industries including banking, insurance, education, and the retail sector. In fact, health care is noticeably behind in its attempts to incorporate digital resources and research. But as a result of the expansion within other industries, there has been a growing demand for people with the knowledge and skills to do this work in health care fields. People with this particular skill are referred to as data scientists, and they are some of the most sought-after specialists these days. As a nation, we have already started to realize the importance of cultivating this ability.

What are the specific skills of a data scientist that have become so coveted by various industries? One is the capacity to understand information technology. Another is the capacity to understand statistics. And a third skill, perhaps most surprising, is the capacity to understand the business side of operations in a given field. It helps to think of health care as an information business: collecting, processing, summarizing, analyzing, and then returning information to patients and doctors. Let's not forget that outcomes, too—mortality rates, rehospitalization rates, postoperative successes—are information.

Currently, educational institutions are not able to produce enough data scientists to serve the demand for them, let alone to serve the rising demand for them in health care fields. As a result, one of the big issues that health care companies are likely to struggle with for a while concerns where we find people who are able to do this kind of work.

What I picture happening is something like this: some of those trained in health care technology will have to be trained in data science, and some of the researchers and statisticians in health care will have to learn the technology side of things in order to fill the current void. The cross-training that I'm suggesting here involves training people who are already experts in one area to become knowledgeable in another. But that will only partly address the issue.

In addition to training people who already have one specialization to acquire another specialization, health care companies must build their own capability. They will need to produce a steady stream of employees trained in multiple fields. For now, however, even though it could become very expensive very quickly, they could subcontract help from companies that are developing the products and services they need. Even health care companies that already use third-party tools and technologies still need to develop basic expertise in-house in order to run, manage, and maintain their specific systems. Continuous monitoring, continuous upgrading, and a keen eye for any hiccups and bugs along the way are necessary capabilities for any organization looking to engage AI on behalf of its patients and physicians.

Physicians' Role

I suggest that in order for knowledge specific to the domain of health care to guide this expansion of resources, physicians will need to take a bigger role in this transformation than they have so far. Physicians *need to become the leaders* of this shift within health care. Ultimately, they should be the ones responsible for the algorithms. This means that physicians must be able to understand, generate, monitor, correct, and refine systems during early development and testing phases, and of course, during implementation. Knowledgeable physicians absolutely need to lead algorithm development teams, and physicians who lead the incorporation of AI into clinical practice will need to train other physicians to *understand* the information conveyed by the machines and *to use* that information in their daily and hourly engagement with patients.

I cannot stress this enough: physicians need to be involved at a very high level in governance and policy development. They must be able to build expertise, including the methodology and materials needed for training other physicians. I want to suggest, too, that the United States put a high priority on developing and refining AI systems and on training and recruiting people with the skills necessary to do that same work well. This is mission critical for the functioning of individual health care companies and for the progress of the health care delivery process as a whole.

Taking the 30,000-Foot View

From the 30,000-foot view, AI and machine learning are best overall at predictive tasks: looking at large amounts of data and predicting diseases, diagnoses, and treatment options, and determining what will work and what will not work. Utilizing these tools for predictive tasks will change, for the better, at least three aspects of the way we approach disease processes.

1. **Efficiency will increase.** This is likely to happen first on the side of clinical science. Physicians will become more efficient at studying data and images. Efficiency will increase, as well, in doctors' offices and in interactions with patients. Finally, there will be greater efficiency on the business side of health care, especially in terms of cost reduction. Most of the efficiencies will be gained where mundane, repetitive tasks are used.

2. **The practice of medicine will change.** Consider specialties that are heavily involved with certain procedures or operations. AI outcomes research, or predictive analytics, might show that one procedure is better than another. That is going to change the practice of medicine in certain special-

ties. In general, the practice of medicine is likely to become less wasteful as doctors can be more and more precise about exactly which patients will be helped by which procedures. There is the potential to decrease the total number of procedures, or even eliminate certain procedures, once data shows that some of them may not be contributing to good outcomes or may even be a detriment to good outcomes. The elimination of wasteful procedures and the potential addition of new and more successful ones will shift the work that is being done by physicians. The tech world actually offers us a model here: companies that have mastered the data, such as Google and Facebook, also have mastery of the field. The same will be true in health care: whichever companies have the most data, have the best data scientists, and can generate great algorithms are going to be the ones that are more successful in the long run, once they set the processes in motion.

3. **The research landscape will also change.** Multiyear processes will be significantly condensed because of the ability of AI to help with all stages of the process, from generating the most reasonable hypotheses to determining the extent to which an intervention actually works. The ability to study retrospective data allows us to generate better conclusions about existing data and better hypotheses for future studies. Additionally, there will be a change in the institutional home of research. To date, academic medical centers have played a central role. But now that patient data is becoming central to research, health care delivery companies that have the data are likely to invest more in that research. Research will become a business imperative; it will be a necessary component of making a company better, both clinically and financially. Companies

will have their own teams to generate research from the populations represented in their data, so their physicians can then make better clinical decisions. Having research talent within an organization will be a deciding factor for success.

These three changes, if they are to occur successfully and become sustainable, require a dramatic shift in the business model of health care. The fee-for-service model is dependent on increasing the number of medical interventions and procedures. We cannot have companies continuing to profit from running more tests, prescribing more drugs, doing more surgeries, and making money off people who are sick. Essentially, the increased ability to predict outcomes will throw light on current processes and potentially eliminate a number of them. This ought to have the effect of shrinking the market. In other words, a volume-based, fee-for-service company will see its potential to make money shrink.

The value-based companies making money by keeping patients healthy will be able to utilize the new technologies to make them even better at what they do. Eliminating waste and pinpointing the best tests and treatment options will enable these companies to offer the biggest bang for the buck and help their patients live healthier lives. *Making money off people's good health rather than off their sickness* is a way for companies to profit while also doing the good that the field of health care was intended to do.

Already there are signs of change in this direction. With payers tightening their purse strings, and with the technology offering solutions, the change to value-based care is likely to happen much faster. Similarly, the move toward involving patients more in their own care will be enhanced greatly by the findings from AI analyses. Doctors are likely to find it easier to involve patients when there is a more solid knowledge base to share about various options for care plans. And since value-based care has a stronger preventive focus, data from AI can be used to give patients a greater role in helping avoid disease. We will see a strengthening of the relationship between having access to predictive knowledge and taking preventive actions that reflect that knowledge.

Focusing on value-based care will decrease the need for phone calls to the doctor and for clinic visits. When a physician can monitor AI systems, track their recommendations, and sign off on them, that physician will be better able to take care of patients remotely. Sore throats, flu, and other everyday ailments can be successfully treated without patients having to travel to the hospital or clinic. What a system like this can do is potentially decrease the need for physical space, decrease some of the need for face-to-face interaction with the physician, decrease the need for other people to be the intermediaries transferring information back and forth between patient and physician, and ultimately, decrease the need for hospital beds.

Privacy and Data Security Concerns

As with any system that utilizes tremendous amounts of data, there are and will be security and privacy concerns. I don't want to discount these concerns. In fact, I believe this is an area that will only grow in importance the more data we are able to collect. There is an argument to be made that streamlining the ways we transmit information will keep it more secure if for no other reason than by reducing the unintended leakage of private data due to human error or resolve. But that argument is usually countered by claims that mass amounts of data are vulnerable to machine error or to hackers and others with malicious intent.

This give and take between sharing data and risking their loss or misuse means that companies will have to come up with much more stringent ways of securing, protecting, and transmitting information. It may be that new AI technologies will develop the ability to secure data much better than we have done so far. But the need to enhance data security remains a significant point of concern and a growing challenge for an industry and practice that will rely more and more on mass amounts of information in order to provide reliable, efficient, and affordable care.

CONCLUSION

Let me share my family story.

Our daughter was born in the early nineties. We had moved that year to a new city, and I had started my first job out of medical training. My wife's pregnancy and delivery were both uneventful. We came home from the hospital and everything was good. But within two or three months of my daughter's birth, I noticed that she was not making eye contact. When I looked into her eyes, she would look away. As the weeks went by, I noticed that she would not smile at me or her mother, no matter how hard we tried to make her smile. I remember thinking that something was wrong. I kept noticing little things in her behavior including certain peculiar movements of her hands and the persistent lack of eye contact. She did not like being out of the house in a social situation and would cry around people, in crowded places especially. When I was in medical school, the symptoms of my daughter's condition were not reviewed in any detail, but I knew she had what sounded like autism. It was devastating!

I remember when we decided to contact the pediatrician to inquire about autism. In those days, doctors would tell you that it was necessary to wait until a child was three years old to diagnose.

So even though, by the time she was about a year old, my wife and I had already figured out that our daughter was autistic, there would be no official diagnosis or intervention until she had turned three years of age. When she did turn three, we took her to a specialist, got the official diagnosis, and began treatment. At the time, applied behavior analysis (ABA) was just beginning to be practiced, and so I connected with researchers at a nearby university medical center to learn more and enrolled our daughter in a program with a company that was offering that treatment near to where we lived.

We were lucky to be able to start our daughter with ABA, a relatively intensive program of thirty to forty hours per week. A therapist would work one-on-one with her, essentially teaching her how to learn. Later, she went to a special school where there were difficulties fitting her into an appropriate class. Her condition was in the moderate range, but the classes that were offered were for kids whose conditions were severe. This made it hard for her to adjust. She finished the special school at age twenty-two and graduated out of the school system. Now she attends a day program from morning until early afternoon, and then she comes home to a program we have set up for her.

As she grew up, we discovered that she had some good fine-motor skills, and we let her experiment with a few activities that require those skills. She's come to enjoy making jewelry.[32] My wife taught her how, and now she has a business: an online shop and a training program that teaches other autistic kids to make jewelry. Our daughter has been able to take care of her own things, with some supervision, and she's a happy kid.

That's our story.

---

32   See my daughter's website, www.designsbysiri.com.

Using AI to Predict, Diagnose, and Treat Autism

My daughter was my first experience, my very first interaction, with an autistic child. I learned a lot from her, far more than I had in my medical training, and more than was available to me in the scientific literature at that time.

Today, there's a lot more research and literature on the topic of autism, but, surprisingly, it is not solid.

What I mean is that our understanding of the condition hasn't changed much in the last twenty to twenty-five years. We don't have the ability to make predictions about the condition. We don't know the risk factors, and we don't have prevention plans. It is true that diagnosis is now done sooner. Instead of waiting until the three-year mark, doctors are diagnosing children at around the age of two and a half, sometimes even sooner. In part, the earlier diagnosis is the result of our knowledge that the sooner we can intervene on behalf of autistic children, the better off they will be overall and the more improved their outcomes will be.

While diagnosis of autism is now done earlier in a child's life, treatment has not changed. It's the same ABA program, critiqued and refined over the years. Although ABA therapy ameliorates symptoms and helps children become capable of growth, no other treatment has been shown to improve the overall condition. Beyond ameliorative treatment, there is nothing even remotely like a cure in sight.

Prevention, diagnosis, and treatment are all further complicated by the fact that children with autism can have other medical problems associated with it. Seizures, for example, are very commonly associated with autism, as is aggressive or self-injurious behavior.

By all accounts, autism is a very complicated condition. There are no blood tests or biomarkers that show anomalies or clearly indicate the condition. The diagnosis itself can be difficult to make, and treatments, as I've noted, are limited. Nevertheless, autism is also the condition with the fastest increasing cost of care. The cost of treating autism spectrum disorder is growing at an annualized rate of 17.6 percent![33]

If we could collect and analyze all the information there is about autism, including medical records, environmental and social information, and the like, we may find some clues about what causes it, and we might be able to say something definitive about it. Let's take a closer look at the three components of health care that we've been discussing in this book—prevention, diagnosis, and treatment—as they relate to the case of autism.

1. *Prevention.* We don't know how to prevent autism, because we don't know its etiology or cause. With autism, only a very, very small percentage of cases can be identified genetically. Prediction is further complicated by the appearance of autism in association with other medical problems. Right now, the association of these conditions is largely a mystery.

   Now, we do know that autism is a developmental disorder, and that the condition starts when the brain is being formed in the womb. This is the case, even though the clinical diagnosis is delayed until after the first few years of life. There are some technologies that have been helpful, such as one that uses AI to review MRI scans and detect autism in very young children. But given that this is a condition that begins in the womb, diagnosis at six months can still seem rather late.

---

33 Joseph L. Dieleman, et al., "US Spending on Personal Health Care and Public Health, 1996–2013," *Journal of the American Medical Association* 316, no. 24 (December 27, 2016): 2627–2646, https://doi.org/10.1001/jama.2016.16885.

And the way we would identify those factors is, of course, by collecting data. In general, our genomic data is good. Medical histories, as well as social and environmental data on the parents, are often easily accessible. Data from the environment may be useful. If you put all these things together, there may be a way to identify risk factors for autism. Predictive capability would help to prepare parents. Especially when a family already has one child with autism, knowing the risk factors before another pregnancy develops, or even being able to determine those risk factors during pregnancy, could help parents be better informed and better prepared.

2. *Diagnosis*. Autism has an incredibly wide spectrum. Its range varies from very mild cases to very severe ones. We are not yet able to tell why some children have mild symptoms and others such severe ones that they're a danger to themselves or others, banging their heads or chewing their fingers, for example. We are far from utilizing AI learning and analysis to help us determine and make predictions about a child's location on that spectrum.

To diagnose autism, there are several characteristics that would need to be measured over time. These include language development, socialization, behaviors, and body movements. There is no easy way to measure these, to give them, say, numerical values, or assess the degree to which each individual child is different from others with the same condition. The phenotypic characteristics of the condition—the way it appears or manifests itself—are very different in different individuals. This is what makes diagnosis so complicated. There's no single test or biomarker that can tell us that someone does or does not have the condition. AI could be utilized either to recognize subtleties within the current diagnostic process, or even relieve that process of some of its complications and streamline diagnostic accuracy.

3. *Treatment.* I've mentioned the possibility that there may be other better treatments yet to be discovered. I've also mentioned that autism is a condition for which there is no cure. It is a lifelong condition, one often associated with early mortality. There have been several studies looking at the gut biome and the influence of bacteria on the symptoms. Dietary changes have been suggested as a way to control symptoms. But there is no definitive evidence-based treatment protocol to cover the various symptoms and disease spectrum. Could AI help us find another treatment besides ABA, a better one? Or could we fine-tune ABA? And could AI one day help us cure those children whose autism severely limits their lives?

My overall point is this: with autism, everything is really still on the table. Prevention, diagnosis, treatment—each of these categories needs attention. If the current science is not able to find the answer, it may be time to look at other and novel approaches. Machine learning and artificial intelligence may be able to throw some light on autism and improve the lives of those affected by it.

A Final Word to Readers

It is true that we have made massive achievements in the fields of medicine and technology and have even done so in fields that are working to forge collaborations between, or combine, the two areas.

But what a still-young technology such as AI does, in all honesty, is present us with an amazing opportunity to shake loose from certain limitations in our knowledge and our practice. It also allows us *to better connect our knowledge with our practice.* Too often, the actual practice of medicine suffers from limitations in knowledge and resources, as well as limitations in time and in the ability to process very large amounts of data. AI and machine learning offer the very assistance we need not only to make breakthroughs in medical science but also to change for the better in the way we go about the day-to-day practice, patient by patient, of delivering quality care.

If we can resist our fear of AI technology, recognize the ways that the technology is useful *to us,* for the purposes *we determine for it,* and if we can develop practitioners and researchers who are able to make informed judgments about how to utilize the technology to its full potential, we are likely to move the overall field of health care in directions that have only been dreamed about.

There are untapped possibilities that AI technology—with its ability to synthesize and analyze currently available data sets and notice the subtlest of details—can help us realize.

In honor of those who would benefit tremendously from the insights provided by AI and machine learning—patients, health care professionals, and the overall system of business interests and investment that supports them—I want to challenge my readers to take up the urgent task of developing the role played by artificial intelligence in clinical practice. Bring to bear your knowledge, skills, and training. Be open to new learning and to cross-training in ways that would allow you to participate in, even lead, the project of tackling and solving our direst health problems. Better health across the country, and across the globe, is in your hands.

ACKNOWLEDGMENTS

I would like to acknowledge all the smart and good people I have worked with over the years in health care, technology, innovation and research areas, who taught me, challenged me, trusted in me, guided me, inspired me and were kind to me.

Thank you to my teammates at CREST Network, Dustin Ballard, Mary Reed, David Vinson, Adina Rauchwerger, Dustin Mark, Mamata Kene and Dana Sax for believing in me and supporting my vision of technology.

And thanks to my supervisors Jason Eiband, Edward Baddour, John Skerry, Karen Murrell, and Tracy Lieu for allowing me the freedom to explore areas of technology, research, and clinical care.

Thanks to all the physicians using the RISTRA platform, contributing to the clinical research mission of CREST Network, and making the vision of a Learning Health System possible.

ABOUT THE AUTHOR

Uli K. Chettipally, MD, MPH, is a speaker, physician, researcher and an innovator. He is passionate about delivering artificial intelligence-enabled solutions to physicians to improve patient outcomes. As the chief technology officer of CREST Network, he designed, developed and implemented a region-wide clinical decision support platform to deliver real-time predictive analytics at the point of care—for which he received the "Pioneer" award for Innovation from Kaiser Permanente. He also received the Morris F. Collin award for his research with his team from The Permanente Medical Group. His other roles include: president of the Society of Physician Entrepreneurs, San Francisco Bay Area chapter; member, board of directors, San Mateo County Medical Association; assistant clinical professor of medicine, University of California, San Francisco. To connect with Dr. Chettipally and learn more about his work, visit InnovatorMD.com.

Printed in the USA
CPSIA information can be obtained
at www.ICGtesting.com
JSHW011449280823
47404JS00009B/471